■ DRUGS
The Straight Facts

Body Enhancement Products

DRUGS The Straight Facts

Alcohol

Antidepressants

Body Enhancement Products

Cocaine

Date Rape Drugs

Designer Drugs

Diet Pills

Ecstasy

Hallucinogens

Heroin

Inhalants

Marijuana

Nicotine

Prescription Pain Relievers

Ritalin and Other Methylphenidate-Containing Drugs

Sleep Aids

■ DRUGS
The Straight Facts

Body Enhancement Products

Thomas M. Santella

Consulting Editor
David J. Triggle
University Professor
School of Pharmacy and Pharmaceutical Sciences
State University of New York at Buffalo

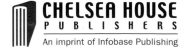
CHELSEA HOUSE
PUBLISHERS
An imprint of Infobase Publishing

Body Enhancement Products

Copyright © 2005 by Infobase Publishing

Chelsea House
An imprint of Infobase Publishing
132 West 31st Street
New York NY 10001

ISBN-10: 0-7910-8197-4
ISBN-13: 978-0-7910-8197-6

Library of Congress Cataloging-in-Publication Data
Santella, Thomas M.
   Body enhancement products/Thomas M. Santella.
      p. cm.—(Drugs, the straight facts)
   Includes bibliographical references and index.
   ISBN 0-7910-8197-4 (alk. paper)
   1. Doping in sports. 2. Anabolic steroids. I. Title. II. Series.
RC1230.S26 2005
362.29—dc22   2004026179

Chelsea House books are available at special discounts when purchased in bulk quantities for businesses, associations, institutions, or sales promotions. Please call our Special Sales Department in New York at (212) 967-8800 or (800) 322-8755.

You can find Chelsea House on the World Wide Web at
http://www.chelseahouse.com

Text and cover design by Terry Mallon

Printed in China

WKT 21C 10 9 8 7 6 5 4 3 2

This book is printed on acid-free paper.

All links and web addresses were checked and verified to be correct at the time of publication. Because of the dynamic nature of the web, some addresses and links may have changed since publication and may no longer be valid.

Table of Contents

The Use and Abuse of Drugs

The issues associated with drug use and abuse in contemporary society are vexing subjects, fraught with political agendas and ideals that often obscure essential information that teens need to know to have intelligent discussions about how to best deal with the problems associated with drug use and abuse. *Drugs: The Straight Facts* aims to provide this essential information through straightforward explanations of how an individual drug or group of drugs works in both therapeutic and non-therapeutic conditions; with historical information about the use and abuse of specific drugs; with discussion of drug policies in the United States; and with an ample list of further reading.

From the start, the series uses the word *"drug"* to describe psychoactive substances that are used for medicinal or non-medicinal purposes. Included in this broad category are substances that are legal or illegal. It is worth noting that humans have used many of these substances for hundreds, if not thousands of years. For example, traces of marijuana and cocaine have been found in Egyptian mummies; the use of peyote and Amanita fungi has long been a component of religious ceremonies worldwide; and alcohol production and consumption have been an integral part of many human cultures' social and religious ceremonies. One can speculate about why early human societies chose to use such drugs. Perhaps, anything that could provide relief from the harshness of life—anything that could make the poor conditions and fatigue associated with hard work easier to bear—was considered a welcome tonic. Life was likely to be, according to the seventeenth century English philosopher Thomas Hobbes, *"poor, nasty, brutish and short."* One can also speculate about modern human societies' continued use and abuse of drugs. Whatever the reasons, the consequences of sustained drug use are not insignificant—addiction, overdose, incarceration, and drug wars—and must be dealt with by an informed citizenry.

The problem that faces our society today is how to break

the connection between our demand for drugs and the willingness of largely outside countries to supply this highly profitable trade. This is the same problem we have faced since narcotics and cocaine were outlawed by the Harrison Narcotic Act of 1914, and we have yet to defeat it despite current expenditures of approximately $20 billion per year on "the war on drugs." The first step in meeting any challenge is always an intelligent and informed citizenry. The purpose of this series is to educate our readers so that they can make informed decisions about issues related to drugs and drug abuse.

SUGGESTED ADDITIONAL READING

David T. Courtwright, *Forces of Habit. Drugs and the Making of the Modern World*. Cambridge, Mass.: Harvard University Press, 2001. David Courtwright is Professor of History at the University of North Florida.

Richard Davenport-Hines, *The Pursuit of Oblivion. A Global History of Narcotics*. New York: Norton, 2002. The author is a professional historian and a member of the Royal Historical Society.

Aldous Huxley, *Brave New World*. New York: Harper & Row, 1932. Huxley's book, written in 1932, paints a picture of a cloned society devoted only to the pursuit of happiness.

David J. Triggle, Ph.D.
University Professor
School of Pharmacy and Pharmaceutical Sciences
State University of New York at Buffalo

1

The History of Body Enhancement Products: Defining the Problem

Since the dawn of competitive sports, athletes have used enhancement drugs and methods to increase their performance and reach artificially heightened levels of athleticism. Although the past century has seen increased regulation and testing for enhancement drugs, it has also seen an equally increased level of use. Today, enhancement drugs are used all over the world, at all levels of sport, from high school athletics to the highest rungs of Olympic competition. These drugs, however, have gone beyond their traditional role as artificial aids for athletes. They are now used by teenagers and adults alike to increase energy, lose weight, and achieve better-looking physiques. This trend has been reinforced by a society that places an extremely high value on "being number one" and having a "perfect body." The trend of body enhancement drug use for sports, however, although it seems to be escalating exponentially, is far from new.

EARLIEST USE

The first evidence of athletes using performance enhancers[1] dates back to the very origins of competitive sports (Figure 1.1). As early

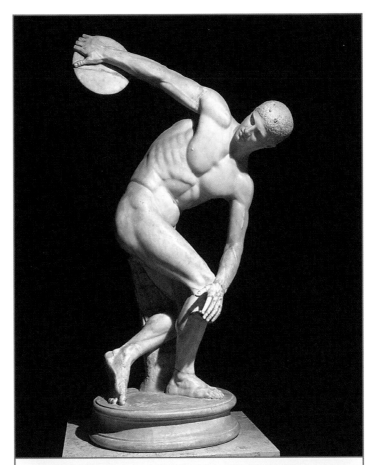

Figure 1.1 Sculpted in the 5th century B.C., Myron's *Discobolus* is regarded as one of the earliest tributes to athletic perfection. Produced in Greece, the meaning of *Discobolus* in modern language is "the disk thrower." The statue exemplifies the flawless anatomy sought by Greek Olympic athletes.

as the 18th Olympiad in 708 B.C.—over 2,700 years ago—long jumpers used hand-held stones called haltcres. These stones, if swung properly, could effectively propel the athlete forward to help increase the distance he jumped. Unlike modern enhancement drugs, haltcres were not only legal but actually encouraged. The ancient Greeks, however, were not entirely innocent in the methods they used to improve performance. They, like today's ultra-competitive athletes, used drugs in sport. Ancient Greek athletes were known to consume strychnine, alcohol, cocaine, and caffeine to increase their endurance during competition. In addition, hallucinogenic mushrooms were used not only by athletes, but also by warriors who needed to "get psyched up" before a battle.

The Greeks were not the only ancient civilization to realize that drugs could serve as a shortcut to athletic success. In ancient Rome, racehorses were given enhancing drugs before races and gladiators often used stimulants before entering the arena. Proof of the extent of the illegal horse-drugging problem is evidenced by the severe punishment meted out to anyone found to have drugged his horse—crucifixion. Despite the severity of punishment for drugging horses, Romans and other people from civilizations around the world had few qualms about drugging themselves—they often took cocaine and caffeine as enhancement products.

MODERN USE

In World War II (1939–1945), both the Germans and the Americans used enhancement drugs in combat. German soldiers were given anabolic-androgen (muscle-building) steroids in order to make them more aggressive. Meanwhile, American soldiers were supplied with amphetamine—a stimulant—so they would need less sleep to stay alert during battle. When American soldiers returned home after the war, some brought with them an insatiable appetite (and often an addiction) for body enhancing drugs that soon spread to the general population.

Experts have assumed that throughout the 20th century, the use of body enhancing drugs was widespread, especially among athletes. Even so, no one knows the full extent to which these drugs were and still are abused because those who use them often go to great lengths to hide their abuse. In light of this fact, the best way to uncover the truth about the magnitude of body enhancement drug use is to examine the efforts and strategies adopted to curb body enhancement drug abuse. Nowhere is this clearer than with respect to the Olympics, the highest level of competitive sporting.

As we have already discussed, athletes have used enhancement drugs such as strychnine, caffeine, heroin, and cocaine for thousands of years. Likewise, before the 20th century, the majority of enhancement drugs used by Olympic athletes were various combinations of these substances. In the early 1900s, two important scientific discoveries were made that changed

BODY ENHANCEMENT DRUGS, IN SO MANY WORDS

Body enhancing drugs have been used for so long by so many people that there are several English words that derive from the practice. The word *assassin* comes from a word that originated in the Middle Ages, *hashshashim*, a name given to certain Muslim warriors during the Crusades. These warriors were known to smoke hashish, a cousin of marijuana, before going into battle. Another group of warriors, these from Norway, were called "the Berzerkers" due to their rather abnormal actions resulting from the use of psychedelic mushrooms. They were said to go into battle only partially clothed and to fight in a rage, more like beasts than men. Today we use the word *berserk* to refer to a person whose actions have become recklessly defiant. The term that is most often used to describe the practice of using drugs to enhance performance, *doping*, came from a form of alcohol used as a stimulant by South African tribes. The beverage was called *dop* and was made from the fermented skins of grapes. *Doping* first appeared in an English dictionary in 1879. Interestingly, these terms are all related not to athletic competition but to the battlefield. As we will see, modern enhancement drug usage stems more from war than from any other factor.

elite sport. In 1927, Fred Koch, an organic chemist at the University of Chicago, first isolated testosterone, the main male hormone and precursor to the production of anabolic steroids. Although amphetamine was first synthesized in Germany in 1887, it was not until the 1930s that scientists found practical uses for drugs containing this substance. Each of these discoveries led to the production of drugs that are used legally and illegally to enhance or stabilize the body.

ENHANCEMENT DRUG CONTROL BEGINS

As new drug classes such as steroids and amphetamines entered the market, the sports community felt the need for the first time to begin regulating and controlling enhancement drug use in order to maintain a fair playing field and protect athletes. In 1928, the International Amateur Athletic Federation (IAAF) became the first sporting organization to ban the use of enhancement drugs, or "doping." Although it was an admirable step to take, neither the IAAF nor any other athletic organization implemented drug testing, which made any serious attempt to stop athletes from using enhancing drugs futile.

As a result, the doping trend continued to escalate. By the 1950s, both Soviet and American Olympic athletes were known to be using enhancing drugs, including male hormones. Although the use of body enhancing drugs among Olympic athletes became increasingly prevalent, serious efforts to control drug use among athletes were not made for another 18 years.

In the 1960s, two deaths resulting directly from doping led to mounting pressure on the International Olympic Committee (IOC) to address the problem. In 1960, Danish cyclist Kurt Jensen collapsed at the finish line and died from an amphetamine overdose. In response to this tragedy, a European committee was set up to address the problem of doping, but it reached no conclusion and took no action. Then, in 1967, Tommy Simpson, the foremost cyclist in Great Britain at the time, died during the Tour de France, the most prestigious non-Olympic cycling competition. Like Jensen, he had taken substances containing amphetamine. The event was televised and people around the world were horrified as they watched Simpson's death take place before their eyes. As a result, the IOC defined and outlawed doping in 1968 and began testing for drug use at the Mexico Olympics that same year (Figure 1.2).

Although more and more athletic organizations followed the example of the IOC and banned doping, the prevalence and use of doping agents has remained rampant. During the 1970s and 1980s, the use of steroids became a particularly serious problem. In 1972, before the IOC prohibited anabolic steroids, one study found that 68% of Olympic athletes admitted to using them. One possible reason for the IOC's failure to ban steroid use may have been that there was no test available to accurately measure the level of steroids in the body. It wasn't until 1974 that a reliable test was invented. Subsequently, steroids were added to the IOC list of prohibited substances in 1976. In the midst of new regulation, however, one of the most serious and far-reaching body enhancement campaigns was already under way.

INSTITUTIONALIZED ENHANCEMENT

Throughout the 1970s and 1980s, the German Democratic Republic (GDR)—at the time, the eastern, Soviet-controlled section of a divided Germany—was engaged in a systematic, state-sponsored body enhancement program. Essentially, athletes were given dangerous enhancement agents as part of their training regimens without their consent or knowledge— in many cases, the athletes were told that the substances were merely "vitamins." Exact figures are unknown but it has been estimated that around 10,000 athletes received enhancement drugs over a period of two decades. The result of the German drug program was huge in terms of Olympic victories. It has been said that the GDR created some of the greatest Olympic

Olympic crackdown on muscle stimulants

In Major League Baseball's stimulant testing last year, 5 to 7 percent of tests were positive. By comparison, less than four-tenths of a percent of tests at the Summer and Winter Olympics since 1968 turned out positive.

Olympic doping cases and the percent of athletes that tested positive

Summer Games

YEAR	HOST CITY	TESTS	POSITIVES	PERCENT
1968	Mexico City	667	1	0.1
1972	Munich	2,079	7	0.3
1976	Montreal	786	11	1.4
1980	Moscow	645	0	0
1984	Los Angeles	1,507	12	0.8
1988	Seoul	1,598	10	0.6
1992	Barcelona	1,848	5	0.3
1996	Atlanta	1,923	2	0.1
2000	Sydney	2,763	11	0.4
	Total	**13,816**	**59**	**0.4**

Winter Games

YEAR	HOST CITY	TESTS	POSITIVES	PERCENT
1968	Grenoble	86	0	0
1972	Sapporo	211	1	0.5
1976	Innsbruck	390	2	0.5
1980	Lake Placid	440	0	0
1984	Sarajevo	424	1	0.2
1988	Calgary	492	1	0.2
1992	Albertville	522	0	0
1994	Lillehammer	529	0	0
1998	Nagano	621	0	0
2002	Salt Lake City	1,922	7	0.4
	Total	**5,637**	**12**	**0.2**

SOURCE: International Olympic Committee

AP

Figure 1.2 Drug testing for Olympic athletes was first implemented at the 1968 Olympics in Mexico City. Since then, the number of drug tests performed at the Olympic Games has fluctuated but the occurrence of positive tests has remained relatively small. Since Olympic drug testing began, fewer than 0.4% of Olympic athletes have tested positive for drugs. This result, however, may not paint a completely accurate picture of the doping situation as a whole, since many athletes take steps to hide their use of body enhancement products.

sports teams in history during this period. In one striking example of the GDR system, no East German Olympic woman had won a gold medal before 1976; but in the 1976 Montreal Olympics, the East German women's swim team won all but two swimming events. The GDR program's victories, however, did not come without a cost. Giving so many drugs to so many athletes led to a myriad of health problems for thousands of East German athletes.

In recent times, enhancement drug abuse has been recognized in countries all over the world. From China to the

United States, new forms of enhancement drugs that cannot be detected have been created and are being used worldwide. Furthermore, star professional athletes such as Sammy Sosa and Mark McGwire have engaged in performance enhancing techniques that are legal but have been highly criticized.[2] Because of the widespread availability of enhancement drugs, both new and old, it is important that athletes, teenagers, and adults understand both the medical benefits and the dangerous effects of body enhancement drugs. This book provides information on the most common enhancement drugs and drug classes that are used today. Because the spectrum of body enhancement drugs is so large, it is important to point out the difficulties that have arisen and the challenges that have been faced in defining what exactly constitutes a body enhancement drug.

WHAT IS A BODY ENHANCEMENT DRUG?

One of the difficulties that regulating organizations have had when developing lists of prohibited drugs or classifying enhancement drugs is how to determine what an enhancement drug really is. Body enhancement drugs are also referred to as "performance enhancing drugs." When an athlete takes these products to acquire supernormal abilities, it is called "doping." The IOC provides the following definition for doping:[3]

> [A]dministration or use by a competing athlete of any substance foreign to the body or any physiological substance taken in abnormal quantity or taken by an abnormal route of entry into the body with the sole intention of increasing in an artificial and unfair manner, his/her performance in competition. When necessity demands medical treatment with any substance which, because of its nature, dosage, or application is able to boost the athlete's performance in competition in an artificial and unfair manner, this too is regarded as doping.

This carefully crafted and rather wordy definition is a good reflection of the complex nature of defining enhancement drugs in general.

In coming up with a definition, several problems arise. One problem is actually determining when a drug can be said to unfairly affect performance. Most cases are clear. It is unlikely that anyone would deny that heroin or cocaine are drugs that significantly manipulate the body and, therefore, should be outlawed by athletic organizations and placed on prohibited substance lists (in fact, these drugs are illegal not only in sports but in most countries in general). Other substances, however, do not cause such obvious responses. For example, should caffeine be classified as a body enhancing drug? Unlike cocaine or heroin, caffeine is found in many perfectly legal foods such as chocolate, coffee, and soda. Actually, the IOC does outlaw caffeine when it is present in the bloodstream at high levels. Beyond caffeine, however, there are many examples of enhancing drugs that are legal and are not outlawed by most athletic organizations. To identify these products, all you would have to do is to walk into a local nutrition store and pick up any of the thousands of products on the shelves. Clearly, not all enhancing drugs are illegal. How, then, do we determine what makes a drug an enhancement product?

Traditionally, there are two criteria used for defining something as a drug: It is a substance controlled by medical experts, or it is a substance known to have clear physiological effects. These criteria, however, do not adequately describe all substances. Take alcohol, for example; it is not controlled by the medical profession, which would suggest that it is not a drug. However, the physiological effects of alcohol are well known, and many people would argue that it is, in fact, a drug. Clearly, not all drugs that affect performance are easily classified.

In addition to deciding whether a substance is actually a body enhancing drug, another complication involves the legal use of substances for legitimate medical conditions. Take, for example, an athlete who has asthma. Should the athlete be allowed to take medications from the beta-2 agonist class (medications that help open the body's airways)? Certain drugs in this class are prohibited by the IOC, but are necessary for treating the athlete's ailment. (Actually, the IOC does allow use of certain prohibited drugs if they are used as a health treatments for a particular condition.) In addition to defining body enhancers, there is also debate over the ethics of using drugs to increase performance—should athletes have the right to use drugs if they understand the dangers and long-term consequences? Is it fair to allow athletes an artificial advantage over those who do not use enhancement drugs? It is clear that there are many problems in defining and regulating body enhancement substances.

WHY DO ATHLETES USE BODY ENHANCING DRUGS?

- The belief that their competitors are taking drugs
- A willingness to do anything to win
- Pressure to succeed from parents, peers, and coaches
- Pressure to succeed from national governments as well as direct state sponsorship
- Financial rewards

There are many reasons that athletes use drugs to aid performance. The main factor is pressure, which comes in several forms. All athletes put pressure on themselves because they have a basic desire to be successful. Additionally, coaches, family, and friends with high expectations can add more pressure. Beyond this, pressure can come from other athletes, spectators, and the media. Because the rewards (both status elevation and financial) are so great, athletes are often willing to go to dangerous lengths to beat their competitors.

Luckily, practically every substance known and on the market today has been heavily researched and its physiological effects accurately documented. As a result, the World Anti-Doping Agency (WADA) has created a list of prohibited substances that is updated regularly. Typically, body enhancement drugs have been separated into five major classes. These classes will be the focus of the next chapter.

2

Enhancement Drug Classes

In the previous chapter, we discussed the strong role of pressure as a factor in a person's decision to use body enhancing drugs. Once the decision is made, however, there are several ways in which drugs can be used to boost performance. Drugs are used to build muscle mass to add strength, to increase oxygen carriers in the body to boost endurance, to mask pain, to stimulate the body or induce weight loss, and to hide the use of other drugs. In this book, enhancement drugs are separated into several groups, or classes, that include:

- Building Muscle Mass

- Increasing Oxygen Delivery

- Stimulants, Relaxants, Weight Control, and Pain

- Nutritional Supplements

- Masking Drugs (to avoid detection through drug testing).

Each class contains many drugs that affect the body in different ways and have different side effects. These classifications are useful for making sense of the vast quantity of enhancement drugs, but they are also somewhat arbitrary, since they are all interrelated. For example, even though masking drugs are presented as a separate class, they are used to hide traces of drugs in all of the other classes. While some of these drugs are synthetic (artificially produced), and others are natural (made in the body), they are all used to deceive the body's natural processes. Each of these classes will be summarized in this chapter and discussed in detail later.

BUILDING MUSCLE MASS

Perhaps the most common reason people use body enhancing drugs is to build or increase muscle mass. Typically, increased muscle mass is gained through the breakdown and rebuilding of muscle tissue. Have you ever felt soreness in your muscles after prolonged exercise or activity? To work properly, your muscles use oxygen to allow you to run, jump, lift, and accomplish many other tasks. When muscles are overworked, muscle tissue (the material muscles are made of) breaks down and causes the soreness that you feel. The soreness is a way to let your body know that it needs to build bigger muscles—and it will! Using protein, your muscles will rebuild themselves to be stronger than they were before. One of the main purposes of exercise is to break down muscle tissue in order to rebuild it and make it stronger. This process, however, is both difficult and time consuming. As a result, some people resort to using drugs that artificially mimic this process but do not require the work, often with dangerous consequences. Perhaps the most common of these are anabolic androgenic steroids.

Steroids

A steroid is one of many hormones used by the body's endocrine system. The body produces hormones to stimulate cells in specific ways. There are several hormones that are classified as steroid hormones. These include testosterone and cortisol in males, and estrogen and progesterone in females. Steroid hormones stimulate either the breakdown of tissue (called a catabolic effect) or the building of tissue (an anabolic effect) by sending a signal that tells bone and muscle cells to increase or decrease protein production. Typically, most users—particularly bodybuilders and other athletes who require size and strength to excel in their sport—take anabolic steroids because they lead to increased muscle mass. These steroids, however, also cause adverse side effects such as liver damage, depression, baldness, and infertility.

Other Muscle Builders

In addition to steroids, there are other drugs used to build muscles. Many of these drugs, like steroids, are hormones that

A NOTE ABOUT HORMONES

Because many body enhancing drugs are made from natural hormones produced by the body, it is important to understand how and where these hormones are originally created. There are more than 20 major hormones produced within the body. A good way to think about hormones is as regulators. Various levels of hormones are distributed throughout the body, reacting to all kinds of environmental and physiological factors. Hormones affect many bodily functions, including growth and development, sexual function, and mood. The system responsible for creating and dispersing these hormones is called the endocrine system.

The endocrine system is made up of glands that make and distribute hormones throughout the body. The hypothalamus, pituitary, thyroid, adrenals, pancreas, ovaries (in females), and testes (in males) are the primary glands of the endocrine system. The pituitary gland is often referred to as the "master gland" because it is the only gland that receives messages directly from the brain. In turn, it sends messages to all the other glands of the endocrine system. The endocrine system is responsible for everything from regulating the level of sugar in your blood to stimulating your growth and adjusting your metabolism (which controls your weight). The endocrine system is crucial for the development and health of your body. Injecting or swallowing hormones can easily disrupt the balance that the endocrine system is designed to maintain.

are found naturally in the body. Examples include human chorionic gonadotropin (hCG), luteinizing hormone (LH), human growth hormone (hGH), and insulin. There are also non-hormone drugs that can cause unnatural muscle growth. Examples include clenbuterol and tertbutaline, which are part of a drug class called beta-2 adrenergic agents. As with steroids, these types of agents can disrupt the body's natural function and cause serious damage to the body.

INCREASING OXYGEN DELIVERY

Some athletes are not necessarily concerned with building muscle mass but instead want to increase their endurance during intense physical activities. Long-distance marathon runners, skiers, and cyclists all must be able to engage in aerobic activity for extended periods of time. The ability to remain highly active over a long period of time is extremely dependent on your body's capacity to deliver oxygen to the areas that need it most. When you run, hike, or bike for a long distance and find yourself gasping for air, it is your body's way of telling you that it needs more oxygen. If your body cannot deliver enough oxygen, you will be unable to continue the activity and will have to stop and catch your breath. Just as muscles can be built through exercise, so too can your body's ability to hold and deliver oxygen be increased through consistent training. But as with muscle growth, some people use methods that unnaturally curb oxygen loss without properly training the body.

Blood doping, or "packing," is a method that has been used to increase the number of red blood cells in the body. Red blood cells are cells within blood that are primarily responsible for collecting and distributing oxygen. When oxygen flows into your lungs, red blood cells pick up the oxygen molecules and take them to the parts of the body where they are needed. Blood doping is the intravenous infusion of whole blood, which includes red blood cells, into a person's bloodstream. The increased number of cells results in increased oxygen delivery and, therefore, greater endurance. In the past, athletes have used both their own blood (extracted at an earlier time and then infused later), and the blood of others.

Blood doping is known to result in drastically increased blood pressure and heart failure. Like putting too much gas in a car, the additional blood strains and adds pressure to the circulation system. In addition, infusing another person's blood is very risky, as it could contain and transfer infectious agents that cause serious diseases, such as human immuno-deficiency virus (HIV) and acquired immunodeficiency syndrome (AIDS). Also, if the wrong blood type is used, problems such as jaundice, blood clots, metabolic shock, and kidney damage can result.

In addition to increasing the amount of blood, there are also protein hormones and artificial oxygen carriers that have been designed to increase the production of red blood cells. Drugs such as erythropoietin (EPO) and artificial hemoglobin have been used to create red blood cells. As with packing, stimulating the production of new red blood cells can result in heart failure.

STIMULANTS, RELAXANTS, WEIGHT CONTROL, AND PAIN

All sports require vast amounts of energy and focus. Using stimulants to heighten concentration and energy levels is a practice as old as sport itself. As we have already discussed, there are many different forms of stimulants. Stimulants include everyday products such as chocolate, coffee, and cola, but there are many more potent stimulants such as amphetamines and cocaine. Athletes may use stimulants because they speed up the heart, which, in turn, speeds up other bodily functions, allowing a runner to run faster, a jumper to jump higher, and a cyclist to ride farther. The side effects of stimulants include nervousness, high blood pressure, and sometimes even sudden heart attack and cardiac death.

Just as some people stimulate their bodies, others use different drugs to become more relaxed. Marijuana, alcohol, and a class of drugs called beta-blockers are all relaxants. You may be asking yourself, "If stimulants make you run faster, wouldn't relaxants make you run slower and, if that is the case, why would anyone want to use them?" Actually, people do not use relaxants to increase their energy level but, as the name suggests, to relax. These drugs have a sedating quality that allows people to temporarily withdraw from the pressures of everyday life. For athletes, these drugs may be particularly

DID YOU KNOW?

Caffeine, a substance found in coffee, tea, chocolate, and cola, is an addictive drug! In fact, caffeine, amphetamines, heroin, and cocaine all affect the same area of the brain. And that's not all—scientists have found that over 90% of Americans consume significant amounts of caffeine every day. Could it be true that over 90% of Americans are addicted to a drug? Fortunately, the effects of caffeine on the body are significantly less dramatic than the effects of stimulants like cocaine, heroin, or amphetamines. Still, caffeine affects the brain by sending a message to increase the firing of neurons, which makes the body produce adrenaline and increases energy— this explains why college students often drink lots of coffee when cramming the night before a test. Coffee can keep you awake and give you energy in the short term, but after the initial "rush," your system becomes depressed and even more tired. The average six-ounce (0.17 liters) cup of coffee contains 100 milligrams of caffeine. The International Olympic Committee (IOC) has not banned caffeine completely but it has placed limits on the amount permitted in an athlete's bloodstream. More than eight regular cups of coffee (or four "talls" from Starbucks®) before competing would be enough to disqualify you from Olympic competition.

inviting, since their jobs can be extremely stressful. The side effects of relaxants are as varied as the drugs that make up the class. Negative side effects include fatigue, memory loss, and brain damage.

Many sports such as rowing, horse racing, and boxing require athletes to meet certain weight requirements. As a result, some athletes use diuretics to artificially control their weight. (Diuretics are substances that cause the body to expel more urine than it normally would, which can lower the body weight through water loss.) The use of diuretics has also infiltrated the general population in the form of diet pills. Although most people view weight loss as a positive action, taking diuretics to control weight can cause dizziness, dehydration, and heart and kidney failure. In addition, diuretics do not eliminate fat. They mainly cause the body to lose water, which will return once the body is rehydrated.

Pain is invariably a part of every sport and every person's life. Fracturing or spraining an ankle, pulling a tendon, or bruising an arm are all unwanted and painful injuries. These injuries are an inescapable part of life and sports. To some extent, we judge athletes on their ability to withstand pain: We look up to the boxer who manages to get up before the referee counts him out. We admire those who can persevere in the face of adversity. For example, as Ernest Hemmingway wrote, "man is not made for defeat. A man can be destroyed but not defeated."[4] Pain, however, is more than a proverbial challenge that a person must strive to overcome; it is your body's way of letting you know that something is wrong, that some part needs to be rested or repaired. But rest and repair do not sell out football games or create amateur tennis champions. As a result, drugs are often used to cover up the pain or "mask" the injury so the athlete can continue to perform.

There are many different types of drugs that can be used to mask pain. Narcotics such as morphine and heroin, anesthetics like those you receive at the dentist's office, and hormones like cortisone can all effectively relieve or eliminate pain. This does not mean, however, that the injury is not still there. That is the problem with pain relievers. All they do is mask pain so you can continue to be active, often doing further damage to already injured body parts.

NUTRITIONAL SUPPLEMENTS

Nutritional supplements are often used to enhance the body's natural mechanisms. Because they are unregulated, nutritional supplements are not generally discussed as body enhancing drugs; however, they are widely used and are an important component of the enhancement spectrum. As such, the subject of nutritional supplements will be explored within this book.

3

Building Muscle Mass and Strength: The Truth About Anabolic Androgenic Steroids

Josh shook his head sadly as the police officer guided Mark—headgear still clinging tightly to the sides of his head—into the back seat of the squad car. Mark was no longer kicking or shouting, but his eyes blazed ferociously and the veins in his neck bulged. Josh stood by, helpless.

This was not how their last state wrestling tournament was supposed to end. From the time they were freshmen, Josh and Mark talked about winning the state tournament in their respective weight classes. Of course, Josh and Mark changed weight classes a few times as they made their journey from freshmen "rookies" to senior varsity co-captains.

As a senior, Josh wrestled all his matches at 125 pounds. Mark started the year wrestling at 130, then a few matches into the season jumped to 135. In his new weight class, Mark lost the only match he'd lose all year—a close, tough match. Mark did not take the loss well, to say the least. On the way home, Mark sulked and talked about how he had just blown any shot he had at a wrestling scholarship.

In the days that followed, Mark seemed to put the loss behind him. His focus on wrestling became more intense than ever—he didn't lose again all season. In fact, Mark set a new school record for pins, even as he again jumped weight classes, from 135 to 140. Some of Mark's wins surprised Josh. Mark usually won his matches by outsmarting and outmaneuvering his opponents; now, more and more he was just outmuscling them.

Josh and Mark always practiced, hit the weight room, and did their running together, and Josh had wondered how Mark was able to improve so much without changing any aspect of his workouts. After Mark's first match wrestling at 140, Josh asked him if he was "on the juice"—meaning steroids. In response, Mark had just flexed his biceps, flashed his tough-guy game face, and laughed.

Mark's wrestling career was soaring, but it seemed to Josh that Mark was pushing himself too hard. Mark frequently complained of headaches and tiredness. When they were in class, Mark's hands would sometimes shake as he held a pen. A few weeks before the state tournament, Josh noticed that Mark's skin color was off and that he was starting to break out. It's just stress, Josh told himself. When their teammates asked Josh what was up with Mark, he told them the same thing: "It's nothing more than stress. He's putting a lot of pressure on himself."

Pressure or no pressure, there was no excusing Mark's behavior that afternoon. As the bleachers filled with spectators, and as wrestlers from high schools across the state awaited the beginning of the tournament, the captain of the Springfield team struck. Looking to psych Mark out for their rematch during the tournament, he slapped a Springfield High School bumper sticker across the back of Mark's uniform as he was stretching. Before anyone could react,

Mark tackled the Springfield captain to the ground and began to pummel him. Coach Whann tried to pull Mark away, and was rewarded for his efforts with a punch in the face and a black eye. It was only with the help of the police officer on hand to oversee tournament security that they were able to drag Mark away, first to the locker room and then to the squad car outside.

A second police officer, holding what Josh recognized as Mark's equipment bag, approached the area near the squad car where Coach Whann was standing. The officer pulled a small box from Mark's equipment bag and held it up for Coach Whann to see. A look of shock crossed the coach's face, a look Josh knew mirrored the expression on his own face. Inside the box, as Josh could see all too clearly, were several small glass vials and several neatly arranged, plastic-encased syringes. Mark had been taking steroids.

WHAT ARE ANABOLIC ANDROGENIC STEROIDS?

Perhaps the most common of all body enhancing drugs are those known as anabolic androgenic steroids (often referred to simply—and erroneously—as "steroids"). In order to understand the term *anabolic androgenic steroids,* we must break down the meaning of each of its parts. *Anabolic* (the opposite of *catabolic*) refers to the building of muscle; it is important to note here that not all steroids are anabolic. Cortisone, for example, is a drug commonly used in sports and given to patients after surgery to reduce inflammation. Cortisone is catabolic because it breaks down rather than builds muscle tissue. The term *androgenic* is a combination of the Greek roots *andro,* meaning "man" or "male," and *genic,* meaning "producing." *Androgenic,* therefore, refers generally to the production of physical and sexual characteristics associated with males, and specifically to the testosterone base of these drugs. Finally, the term *steroid* refers to these drugs' classification as hormones. So, an anabolic androgenic steroid (AAS) is essentially a hormone (either synthetic or natural) that builds muscle by mimicking or increasing male-producing characteristics.

Although not all steroids are anabolic, all anabolic steroids *are* androgenic. In other words, there is no AAS that will build muscle without also producing dangerous and unwanted androgenic side effects. In addition, an AAS is only effective when combined with rigorous training (you cannot gain muscle by using steroids and proceeding as a couch potato). Though there are more than 20 forms of anabolic androgenic steroids, they are all derivatives of testosterone, the main male hormone. Because all anabolic androgenic steroids are testosterone derivatives, they all create hormonal imbalances in the body that in turn lead to a host of unwanted side effects. Before moving on to a discussion concerning how anabolic androgenic steroids work, there are three important things to remember about AAS products:

1. Anabolic androgenic steroids do stimulate muscle growth and increase strength.

2. This growth *only* occurs when combined with rigorous physical training.

3. *All* anabolic androgenic steroids cause severe side effects.

HOW DO ANABOLIC ANDROGENIC STEROIDS WORK?

Anabolic androgenic steroids are essentially derivatives of testosterone. Testosterone (Figure 3.1) is a hormone mainly produced in the male testes but also produced in female ovaries (in much smaller quantities) and in the adrenal glands of both sexes. Testosterone is responsible for the development of many important functions in growing people, including skeletal/muscle growth and sexual function. As previously discussed (see Box on page 21), the pituitary or "master" gland

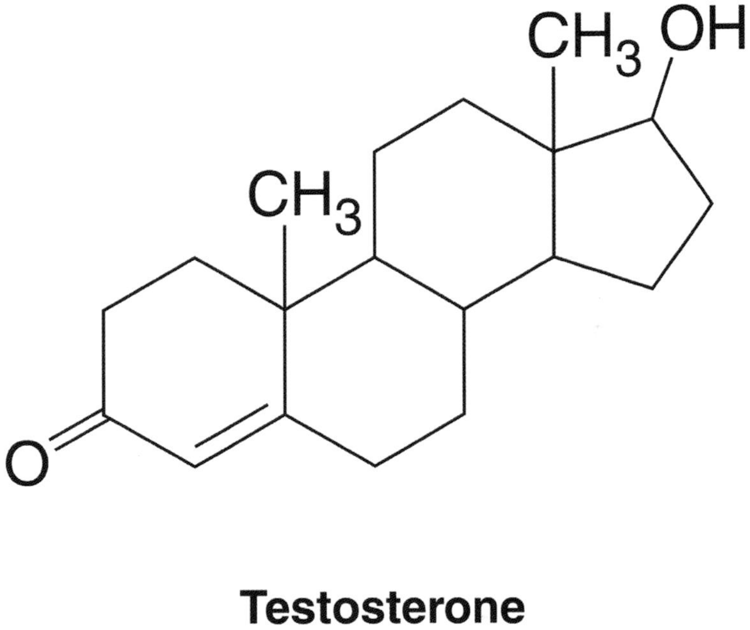

Testosterone

Figure 3.1 The testosterone molecule (illustrated here) is one of the most important chemicals in the bodies of both men and women. Its structure is derived from the 4-ring cholesterol molecule but has additional compounds attached to its rings. Different forms of testosterone result from varying attached compounds.

controls the production of testosterone. In males, the testes are primarily responsible for actually making the hormone. Normally, the pituitary gland senses the level of testosterone in the body and makes adjustments accordingly, in a negative feedback mechanism. That is, if there is too much testosterone, the pituitary gland shuts down production, whereas if the body needs more testosterone, the pituitary gland increases production (Figure 3.2). The use of anabolic androgenic steroids affects the careful equilibrium that usually exists in

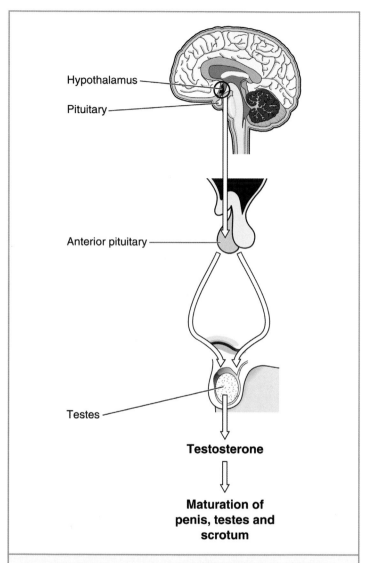

Hypothalamus

Pituitary

Anterior pituitary

Testes

Testosterone

**Maturation of
penis, testes and
scrotum**

Figure 3.2 The production of testosterone in males takes place in the testes (ovaries in females) and is critical in determining the development of many of the body's functions. The pituitary, or "master," gland controls the level of testosterone production. The use of anabolic androgenic steroids significantly compromises the pituitary's ability to regulate testosterone production.

the body by bypassing the pituitary gland's negative feedback system altogether. As we will see, this can cause a number of adverse effects.

AAS can be taken in two ways: orally (in a pill or capsule form) or by injection (oil-based or water-based). When a pill is swallowed or an injection is taken, the synthetic testosterone is absorbed directly into the bloodstream and from there into various cells. These cells have receptors that recognize the testosterone and are programmed to respond to it in certain ways. Steroids work by traveling through muscle cell membranes and connecting to hormone receptors, which are located both in the cell plasma and the cell nucleus. Once the receptor binds to the steroid, it is able to attach itself to the deoxyribonucleic acid (DNA) within the nucleus (Figure 3.4). The DNA contains the genetic information necessary for the organization and function of most living organisms. Once attached to the DNA, the steroid instructs the cell to form a new protein. When muscle cells receive AAS (testosterone), the production of muscle protein is stimulated, resulting in the anabolic effect that causes increased muscle mass and strength. Other cells, however, also receive the testosterone and carry out different functions, such as hair growth and the deepening of the voice, among others. The artificially increased levels of testosterone in the body cause various short-term side effects. With extra testosterone in the body, the pituitary gland shuts down the process of testosterone production, leading to long-term effects such as prostate gland enlargement and psychological problems, including violent mood swings and overaggression.

TYPES OF ANABOLIC ANDROGENIC STEROIDS

There are more than 20 different forms of anabolic androgenic testosterone (Table 3.1), which can be separated into three classifications: C-17 alkyl derivatives of testosterone, esters of 19-nortestosterone, and esters of testosterone. An alkyl is an

FROM CHAMPION TO CRIMINAL IN 9.79 SECONDS!

The gun sounds and the runners take off! They have trained their entire lives for this moment and it will come down to a difference of a hundredth of a second between the glory of winning the gold medal and taking the sad ride home. It is the 1988 Olympics in Seoul, Korea. The contest is being referred to as "the greatest race in history." The crowd is clearly excited as the runners sprint down the 100-meter (109-yard) track. Canadian sprinter Ben Johnson (Figure 3.3) crosses the finish line in 9.79 seconds. He has won the gold medal, broken the world record, and is exalted as the fastest human being on the planet! Three days later, Johnson tests positive for steroid use—and is stripped of his gold medal.

Ben Johnson rose to the pinnacle of his career and quickly lost it all to steroids. Not only did Johnson lose his 1988 gold medal, but he also lost his right to compete in sports and, perhaps worst of all, he lost his pride. It was eventually discovered that Johnson had been abusing steroids for over six years with the full knowledge and assistance of his coach and team physician. Johnson's story shed light and attention on the ever-increasing problem of performance enhancement among athletes. Although Johnson's story may be the most infamous, it is certainly not the only case of a high-profile athlete being connected to steroids. Many other well-known athletes have been connected to or accused of steroid use since the 1988 Olympics, and if history is any guide, there will surely be many more exposed in the years to come.

Source: BBC News. Available online at *http://news.bbc.co.uk/onthisday/hi/ witness/september/24/newsid_3114000/3114220.stm*.

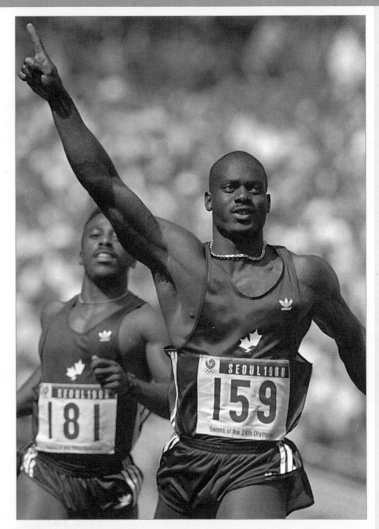

Figure 3.3 *On September 24, 1988, Ben Johnson (pictured here, in front) set a new world record for the men's 100-meter race with a time of 9.79 seconds. Subsequently, Johnson tested positive for steroids and had his gold medal as well as his future in sports taken away.*

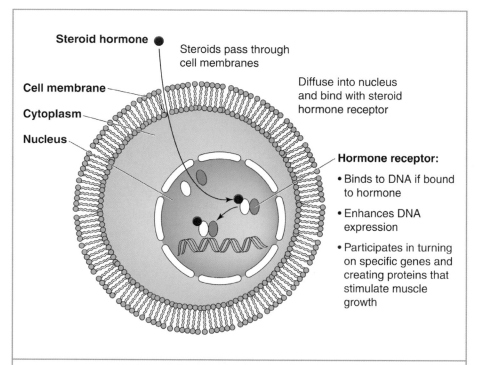

Steroid hormone

Steroids pass through cell membranes

Cell membrane

Diffuse into nucleus and bind with steroid hormone receptor

Cytoplasm

Nucleus

Hormone receptor:

- Binds to DNA if bound to hormone

- Enhances DNA expression

- Participates in turning on specific genes and creating proteins that stimulate muscle growth

Figure 3.4 Once injected or swallowed, the anabolic androgenic steroid hormone passes through the cell membrane and moves directly toward the cell's nucleus, as is illustrated here. Attaching to a hormone receptor, the steroid hormone binds to DNA and instructs muscle cells to produce muscle protein. In other types of cells, different instructions, such as the growth of hair, are carried out.

organic compound derived from methane that is made of carbon and hydrogen, and an ester is a compound that is formed by the reaction between an acid and an alcohol with the elimination of water. From a structural standpoint, the testosterone molecule is a derivative of the cholesterol molecule, with the same four rings, but also has three additional compounds attached to the side of the molecule. Differences between the types of testosterone involve variations in these additional compounds. The C-17 alkyl derivatives have an added alkyl group, the esters have an ester compound attached, and the 19-nortestosterones are missing a hydrogen atom. The differences between these classifications may be subtle; however, because there are varying degrees of danger associated with each, it is important to understand these differences.

The distinguishing factor that characterizes the C-17 alkyl derivatives of testosterone is that they can be taken orally, in pill form. The fact that the C-17 alkyl class of anabolic androgenic steroids is comparatively easy to take makes them particularly popular among athletes. One of the most used AAS, methandrostenolone, or, as it is more commonly referred to, Dianabol or simply D-bol, is a member of this class. In addition to being orally active, the C-17 alkyls also have a relatively short clearance time of 3 to 4 weeks. Clearance time is the amount of time that it takes for a drug to completely leave the body, making it undetectable by a drug test. In other words, if an athlete is abusing D-bol but knows that he or she will be tested, the athlete can stop taking the drug four weeks before the test and most likely pass. It is important to note here that clearance times are not 100% accurate. Other factors, such as a person's weight and rate of metabolism, can affect the clearing time significantly.

STREET/SLANG TERMS FOR STEROIDS

Arnolds

Gym Candy

Juice

Pumpers

Stackers

Weight Trainers

Source: Available online at *http://www.whitehousedrugpolicy.gov/drugfact/ steroids/index.html#production.*

Table 3.1 Types of Anabolic Androgenic Steroids

ORAL ANABOLIC STEROIDS	INJECTABLE ANABOLIC STEROIDS
• Anadrol (oxymetholone)	• Anatrofin (stenobolone)
• Anavar® (oxandrolone)	• Bolfortan (testosterone nicotinate)
• Dianabol (methandrostenolone)	• Deca-Durabolin® (nandrolone decanoate)
• Maxibolin® (ethylestrenol)	• Delatestryl® (testosterone enanthate)
• Methyltestosterone	• Depo-Testosterone (testosterone cypionate)
• Primobolin® (Methenolone)	• Dianabol (methandrostenolone)
• Winstrol® (stanozolol)	• Durabolin® (nandrolone phenpropionate)
	• Enoltestovis (hexoxymestrolum)
	• Equipoise® (boldenone—veterinary)
	• Primobolin (Methenolone)
	• Sustanon 250 (a mixture of testosterone esters)
	• Therabolin
	• Trophobolene
	• Wintrol V (stenozolol—veterinary)

Source: Strauss, Richard H. *Drugs & Performance in Sports.* Philadelphia: W.B. Saunders Company, 1987, p. 61.

The distinguishing characteristic of the esters of 19-nortestosterone is that they are oil-based and must be injected directly into a person's fat reserves. More specifically, esters of 19-nortestosterone are dissolved in vegetable oil and injected for gradual release into extracellular fluid. Because of this, the drug is released at a slower rate over a much longer period of time, which diminishes the harmful androgenic side effects. The most common ester of 19-nortestosterone is nandrolone, also called Deca-Durabolin or just Deca. Because members of the ester of 19-nortestosterone class are stored in the body and released slowly, their clearance times are significantly longer, approximately 6 to 8 months. Although the drugs in this class are generally more effective in terms of their anabolic effect, long clearance times and increased drug testing have led to decreased use of the 19-nortestosterone group.

The final classification, the esters of testosterone, is considered the most dangerous of all AAS. The esters of testosterone are actually derivatives of testosterone that can be either taken orally or injected. Because the drugs in this class so closely resemble natural testosterone, the unwanted androgenic effects—including increased body hair growth and stunted growth of bones—are the most common. The esters of testosterone are popular, however, because a drug test cannot tell the difference between these synthetic forms of testosterone and the natural testosterone that is already in the body. As a result, officials have had to design different testing methods to determine whether these drugs have been used.

Although all forms of AAS have been used by athletes and those who want to "bulk up," the advancement of drug testing and the increased scrutiny of the use of drugs among athletes has actually led to an increase in the use of the most dangerous forms of AAS. Because the esters of 19-nortestosterone (which, by comparison, are the least dangerous) have such a long clearance time, their use has lessened over the years. Conversely, the use of esters of testosterone (the most dangerous form of AAS) has increased because of their comparatively quick clearance times. In addition, users have become increasingly sophisticated and many engage in a process called "stacking." Stacking refers to the practice of combining different AAS in various cycles of use. Most experts today agree that users tend to take a higher quantity of AAS than is necessary to achieve the desired effect. In this case, more is certainly not better. Instead, the more AAS a person uses, the more harmful the side effects will be. With this in mind, we turn next to the important matter of side effects.

SIDE EFFECTS OF ANABOLIC ANDROGENIC STEROIDS

The side effects of anabolic androgenic steroids have been well studied and are well documented. These side effects are very real, very serious, and should not be ignored. In the past, athletes have shrugged off medical testimony regarding these severe side effects, considering them a "scare tactic" that exaggerated the negative side effects while downplaying the positive effects in order to discourage steroid use. But the dangers of AAS use cannot be overstated. Reports of the dangers of AAS use are *not* a scare tactic. The side effects are all too real and should be well understood by anyone who might consider trying to build muscle strength through the use of body enhancement products.

Jaundice and Liver Damage

The liver is adversely affected by the use of AAS. This is because these drugs pass through the liver where they are broken down so the body can dispose of them, and this overworks the liver. The added stress on the liver can lead to jaundice, a condition that causes a yellowing of the skin, tissues, and bodily fluids, and is especially noticeable in the whites of the eyes. Though injectable forms of steroids may still go through the liver, they are generally considered less harsh on the liver than the pill

SIDE EFFECTS OF ANABOLIC ANDROGENIC STEROIDS

- Acne: serious cystic types that leave permanent scars on the face and body.

- Nervous tension, aggressiveness, and psychotic states; paranoia and antisocial behavior.

- Increased sex drive after initial use, but decreased sex drive with repeated use.

- Breast development in males (permanent), also known as gynecomastia.

- Gastrointestinal and leg muscle cramping.

- Headaches, dizziness, and high blood pressure.

- Burning and pain while urinating.

- Testicular or scrotal pain.

- Premature male baldness.

- Excessive body and facial hair growth among women.

- Atrophy (shrinkage) of the testicles and decreased sperm production.

- Prostate enlargement, making urination difficult.

- Enlargement (irreversible) of the clitoris, the female organ analogous to the male penis.

- Disruption of the menstrual cycle.

- Deepening of the voice (permanent for women).

- Stunted growth among adolescents, due to premature stoppage of bone growth.

- Liver damage and jaundice.

Source: Voy, Robert, and Kirk D. Deeter. *Drugs, Sport, and Politics.* Champaign, IL: Human Kinetics Publishers, 1991, p. 24.

forms, because products that pass through the stomach are directly filtered by the liver.

Cardiovascular Problems

Research has indicated that one of the long-term effects of AAS use is lower levels of high-density lipoprotein (HDL) cholesterol (good cholesterol), which helps keep arteries clear. Reductions in HDL cholesterol levels can lead to increased buildup of materials in the blood vessels (plaques), which in turn can result in a variety of heart and vascular problems, such as high blood pressure, atherosclerosis, and heart attack.

Psychological Effects

Testosterone plays an important role in maintaining a person's psychological balance, in both men and women. It is responsible for maintaining an appropriate level of aggressiveness that helps athletes to compete. As you would expect, the overconsumption of testosterone causes unhealthy levels of aggression that cause multiple social problems, including extreme overaggressiveness, often referred to as "roid rage." In addition, depression, psychosis, delirium, suicidal tendencies, mania, and homicidal tendencies have all been linked to AAS use. Often, relationships with loved ones and friends are significantly strained. The abuser may or may not make the connection to steroid use, depending on his or her knowledge of the drug.

EFFECTS AMONG MEN
Sexual Dysfunction

Testosterone is the main male hormone, and too much of it leads to a myriad of unpleasant sexual side effects in men. Although testosterone use initially increases sex drive, it eventually causes the sex drive to fall below normal. This is because the natural testosterone that is produced in the body is being replaced by the synthetic testosterone. Effects such as the shrinking of the testes, the enlargement of the prostate, and the production of sperm with abnormal shapes and reduced function have all been attributed to AAS use.

Premature Baldness and Acne

Research has shown that premature baldness is likely to occur in men who use AAS. A specific metabolite of testosterone called dihydrotestosterone (DHT) causes male pattern baldness by binding to receptors in the scalp and causing the hair follicles to become smaller and less active. A man using AAS accelerates this process by adding more testosterone, and thus more DHT, to his body. Although AAS have not been proven to directly cause baldness, certain forms of AAS speed up the hair loss process in both men and women.

Severe cases of acne have also developed in many users, because AAS cause oil-producing glands in the skin (sebaceous glands) to overproduce natural skin oils, increasing the likelihood that the oils will trap dirt, clog the pores, and become inflamed and infected. The risk of premature baldness and acne are increased if the AAS user has a family history of these conditions.

Gynecomastia

Some men who use AAS develop gynecomastia, the excessive development of breasts, an obviously unwanted effect among athletes who wish to be more "macho." Breast development does not occur for all users but, when it does, the effect is permanent. As a result, many male AAS users have undergone surgical procedures to remove the superfluous breast tissue.

EFFECTS AMONG WOMEN

Testosterone and its counterpart, the female hormone estrogen, are responsible in many ways for determining the sex differences between men and women. As a result, women who take synthetic forms of testosterone develop various male characteristics such as hair growth and a deepening of the voice. These side effects are permanent. In addition, many of the same effects that occur in men occur in women—such as increased aggressiveness and acne. The long-term effects of AAS among women are believed to be the same as for men.

EFFECTS AMONG ADOLESCENTS

One very important effect that occurs among teenage boys who use AAS is stunted growth of muscles and bones. Though the short-term use of AAS may cause the adolescent to gain muscle mass and generally get "bigger," the long-term effect is quite the opposite. When abnormal testosterone levels are present in young men, the natural production of testosterone will be stopped early. This means that the natural growth of the boy's muscles and bones will stop short of their full potential. Simply put, the adolescent will end up being shorter and weaker in the long term than he would have been if he had not used AAS.

OTHER DRUGS USED FOR THEIR ANABOLIC EFFECT

Whereas anabolic androgenic steroids are the most commonly used body enhancement drug, a number of other drugs are also used to synthetically build muscle mass and strength.

Human Chorionic Gonadotropin (hCG)

Human chorionic gonadotropin (hCG) is a naturally occurring hormone that is produced by women when they are pregnant. hCG is not synthetic testosterone: rather, it instructs the body to produce extra testosterone. hCG is a glycoprotein hormone made of two subunits connected by an ionic bond. Combined, the subunits are made up of a chain of 237 amino acids. Interestingly, although the IOC bans hCG for men, it is not banned for women because it may be present in a woman's system if she is pregnant. Additionally, it has no muscle-building capability for women. For men, the use of hCG is relatively infrequent because of its high cost (hCG must be extracted from the urine of a pregnant woman). The side effects of hCG in men are the same as those produced by AAS.

Luteinizing Hormone (LH)

Luteinizing hormone is a naturally occurring hormone that regulates testosterone production in men and converts testosterone to estrogen in women. In men, an increase in LH results in a rise in testosterone levels. The structure of LH is very similar to that of hCG. Like hCG, LH is a glycoprotein and only differs in the number and order of amino acids. The side effects of LH have not been adequately studied and are therefore unknown (they can, however, be assumed to be similar to those for AAS).

Mechanism of Action: LH and hCG

The way that LH and hCG work in the body is very similar to the way anabolic steroids work. LH and hCG are hormones and, therefore, pass through cell membranes and attach to specific hormone receptors. LH and hCG work by targeting Leydig cells, which are located in the testes and are responsible for the production of testosterone. Once in the cell, LH and hCG bind to receptors, attach to DNA strands, and instruct the cell to make more testosterone.

Human Growth Hormone (hGH)

Human growth hormone (hGH) is a naturally occurring hormone that is responsible for general body growth in both men and women. hGH helps the body produce protein while breaking down fat deposits. Too much hCG results in increased muscle mass. Human growth hormone has many legitimate medical uses and is increasingly being used by athletes because it is very hard to detect. The side effects of hCH include acromegaly (overgrowth of hands, feet, and some facial features), enlarged organs, and cardiovascular problems.

Mechanism of Action: hGH

Human growth hormone is a protein hormone normally synthesized by the pituitary gland. It is a continuous chain of 191 amino acids. hGH has both direct and indirect effects on the body. hGH directly affects the production of skin, muscle, and bone cells by targeting specific hormone receptors in each and instructing cells to reproduce. It also targets and breaks down fat cells, which stimulates a person's overall metabolism. In addition, hGH indirectly affects growth by signaling the liver to produce insulin-like growth factor-1 (IGF-1). IGF-1 is a hormone that targets and affects almost every cell in the body. The mechanism of action of IGF-1 is very similar to that of hGH.

LOUISE NUTTALL-HALLIWELL: DEATH OF SCOTLAND'S STRONGEST WOMAN

Her career brought her bodybuilding and powerlifting titles. She competed in Miss Universe competitions. Upstart bodybuilders wanted her as their personal trainer. But for Louise Nuttall-Halliwell, the young bodybuilder once known as Scotland's strongest woman, it took only an overdose of insulin to turn a successful career and bright future into tragedy.

Nuttall-Halliwell collapsed in her home in April 2002 and shortly thereafter fell into a coma that would last two years and end with her death in December 2003, at the age of 38. Although details surrounding Nuttall-Halliwell's death have not been released, quantities of insulin were believed to have been found in her home and at her gym at the time of her collapse. Investigators attributed Nuttall-Halliwell's death to brain injuries consistent with those that would be expected to result from an insulin overdose.

Source: Wilson, Mike. "How Search for Perfect Physique Led To Scottish Bodybuilder's Death." *The Scotsman* (April 14, 2004). Available online at *http://thescotsman.scotsman.com/index.cfm?id=428682004.*

Beta-2 Adrenergic Agonists

Used clinically to help asthma patients, beta-2 agonists relax smooth muscle tissue in the lungs. When injected into the bloodstream, however, these agents are believed to produce an anabolic effect. Typically, beta-2 agonists are taken by asthma patients through inhalers. Once in the lungs, the beta-2 agonist enters muscle cells through beta-2 receptors and sends a signal to relax, which opens up the airway and helps the person breathe more freely. The use of beta agonists by athletes with asthma is legal to help them breathe but illegal for enhancement purposes. An athlete using a beta agonist for a legitimate medical condition must present a physician's note to the proper gaming authority. The side effects of beta agonists include muscle cramps, rapid heartbeat, nausea, headaches, and dizziness.

Insulin

Insulin is a natural protein hormone that helps the body break down sugars, starches, fats, and proteins. Insulin is made of two peptide chains and consists of 51 amino acids. Injected insulin is critical for type 1 diabetes patients, whose bodies cannot make or use insulin properly. Throughout the body, there are many cells that have insulin receptors embedded in their cell membranes. Because insulin helps the cell break down glucose, it improves metabolism. When combined with hGH, insulin can have an anabolic effect, breaking down glucose while also promoting growth. Side effects include nausea, weakness, and shaking. The IOC prohibits insulin unless it is being used for legitimate medical purposes, such as the treatment of type 1 diabetes.

4

Increasing Oxygen

You have probably heard stories or seen movies about a monster, warrior, or vampire that drinks blood, but have you ever heard of professional athletes using blood to increase performance? In fact, the practice of influencing athletic performance by using blood to increase oxygen levels is becoming more and more common among athletes (although none of them actually drinks blood!). This practice of increasing oxygen levels through the use of blood, called blood doping, is defined by the World Anti-Doping Agency as "the use of autologous, homologous, or heterologous blood or red blood cell products of any origin, other than for legitimate medical treatment" and "the use of products that enhance the uptake, transport or delivery of oxygen, e.g. erythropoietins, [and] modified hemoglobin products." (Erythropoietins are chemicals that stimulate the body to produce blood. Hemoglobin is the part of red blood cells that helps carry oxygen through the blood.) Simply put, blood doping is the use of blood, or substances that produce blood, to enhance performance.

How do athletes use blood to enhance performance? There are several ways. These include the infusion of actual blood, the use of erythropoietin, and high-altitude training. Before exploring each of these techniques, we must take a brief detour into the world of hematology (the study of blood).

OXYGEN AND THE BODY

As you probably know, oxygen is absolutely essential for life. The heart and circulatory system are responsible for delivering oxygen throughout the body. This is an amazing system: In just one day, your blood travels nearly 12,000 miles; in one year, your heart beats about 35 million times, and over a lifetime, your heart pumps a million barrels of blood.[5] For the athlete, the amount of oxygen that he or she can process and the time it takes for this oxygen to be delivered to the parts of the body that need it most play a major role in determining performance. Because the difference between winning and losing at the professional level often comes down to just a fraction of a second, even a slight boost in your body's ability to accept oxygen can lead to an athletic victory.

The way the body receives and uses oxygen is quite simple. The major component in the body's oxygen system is the red blood cell (RBC). Red blood cells make up about 40% of the 10 pints of blood in the average human body. Men have an average of 5.2 million RBCs per cubic milliliter, whereas females have 4.6 million. Red blood cells are made in the bone marrow and live an average of 120 days, at which time the liver and kidneys remove them. In addition to RBCs, blood contains white blood cells and plasma. These white blood cells are not involved in the delivery and use of oxygen.

When you breathe in, the oxygen molecules in the air flow into your lungs. At the same time, blood flows through the lungs and the RBCs collect the oxygen molecules. This can happen because each RBC contains hemoglobin, which actually grabs onto the individual oxygen molecules (hemoglobin is made of iron and gives blood its red color). Once the RBC has latched onto the oxygen (each hemoglobin can take 4 oxygen molecules and each RBC is about 33% hemoglobin), it delivers it throughout the body.

Runners, cyclists, and all competing athletes need to have high endurance levels and must use a lot of oxygen and become highly efficient in using oxygen. For example, Lance Armstrong,[6] the champion bicyclist, has a heart that is larger than average and is therefore able to pump more oxygen-rich blood throughout his body. The efficiency of the oxygen system is increased naturally through exercise, but modern athletes are using techniques and drugs that artificially boost RBC levels in the hope of achieving heightened endurance levels.

TYPES OF BLOOD DOPING

Perhaps the simplest form of blood doping is breathing pure oxygen. Perhaps you have seen the popular television series *ER*, where patients are often seen strapped to oxygen masks. The use of oxygen in athletic competition is legitimate and is used often for injured athletes. Studies have shown that, although breathing pure oxygen is useful for medical purposes, it gives no real advantage to athletes. There are other methods, however, that do increase performance.

Infusion

Perhaps the oldest form of unethical blood doping is the infusion of blood. In this simple process, an athlete injects blood into his or her own body, thereby increasing his or her total amount of blood. With more blood and, more importantly, more red blood cells, the athlete is able to accept and use more oxygen at a quicker pace. As a result, the muscles are able to work harder and longer before they get tired, which increases the athlete's endurance.

There are two main forms of infusion. The oldest, called homologous blood doping, is when an athlete accepts blood from another person (usually a relative) and adds it to his or her system just before an athletic competition. Although this tactic is effective in increasing performance, this form of doping, because it involves using blood from other people, comes with a high risk of contracting infectious diseases such as HIV/AIDS and hepatitis. In addition, problems such as jaundice, blood clots, metabolic shock, and kidney damage can develop if the wrong blood type is used. As a result, athletes do not generally favor homologous doping, and there has been a shift toward autologous blood doping.

Autologous doping, like homologous doping, involves the infusion of blood into the body. The difference is that with autologous doping, the athlete takes out some of his or her own blood (about 2 pints out of a total 10 pints in the body) about 10 weeks prior to competition. By the time of the event, the athlete's blood level has most likely returned to normal. Meanwhile, the extracted blood has been frozen and centrifuged (separated into its component parts: white blood cells, red blood cells, and plasma). Just before the event, the athlete injects just the red blood cell portion of the blood extracted earlier, thereby increasing the total amount of red blood cells and the body's ability to process oxygen.

Besides the potential risk of transmitting diseases such as HIV/AIDS, there are two additional possible complications related to blood doping. The first deals with blood's resistance to flow (viscosity). The body's circulatory system is built to handle 10 pints of blood. When athletes blood dope, they add about 2 pints beyond the normal maximum, thereby increasing the total level to about 12 pints. The addition of this new material thickens the blood, giving it a consistency like syrup. The thickened blood causes the possibility of clogging arteries. Just like the plumbing in a house, if there is too much extra material in the pipes, pressure builds up and the pipes get clogged. Left unchecked, the pipes will eventually burst. The added blood has a very similar effect on the body.

The second problem that blood doping causes deals with increased blood pressure. Because the blood is thicker and there is more of it, it becomes more difficult for the heart to push all that blood around. As a result, the heart must work much harder, increasing the potential for and risk of heart failure.

Even with the risk of serious medical problems and despite the possibility of death, some athletes continue to use these blood doping methods. The reason, as studies indicate, is that the extra red blood cells can help increase endurance by more than 20%, which gives the athlete a decided advantage.

Erythropoietin (EPO)

Another form of blood doping involves the injection of a substance called erythropoietin, or EPO. EPO is a natural hormone made by the body, usually secreted by the kidney when the body is low on oxygen (Figure 4.1). It is a glycoprotein hormone made up of 165 amino acids. EPO is responsible for regulating the production of red blood cells. With recent advances in biotechnology, scientists have been successful in creating EPO synthetically. EPO is used legitimately to help certain conditions such as anemia, in which red blood cell production is too low. Like other protein hormones, EPO works by targeting specific cells, in this case, bone marrow stem cells. It attaches to its specified receptor and instructs the cell to produce more red blood cells.

The use of EPO by a person with normal blood production is extremely dangerous. Athletes use EPO because it has the same effect as autologous blood doping, increasing performance. The major difference between the two, however, is that autologous blood doping, while dangerous, is a short-term procedure (blood levels return to normal soon after the additional blood is injected). When EPO is injected, the body loses control of red blood cell production completely. As a result, the blood may become much thicker with EPO than with autologous or homologous doping. The effects of this thickening are the same as they are for infusion but are considered even more perilous because of the lack of control.

High-Altitude Training

The final and most benign form of blood doping is high-altitude training. As the name suggests, some athletes train at high altitudes in order to gain a competitive advantage. The theory behind high-altitude training is that at high altitudes (where there is less oxygen in the air), a person must get used to the lack of air to function. After training under these

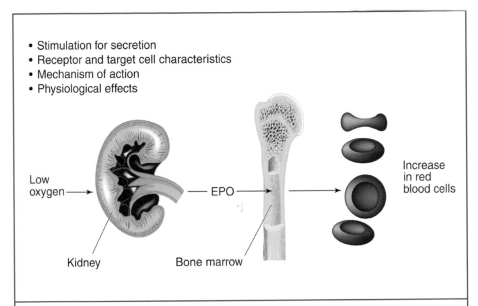

- Stimulation for secretion
- Receptor and target cell characteristics
- Mechanism of action
- Physiological effects

Low oxygen → — EPO → → Increase in red blood cells

Kidney   Bone marrow

Figure 4.1 The production of erythropoietin (EPO) takes place in the kidney during reduced oxygen situations. When the body needs additional oxygen, the kidney secretes EPO, which enters the bone marrow where red blood cells are produced. This increases the production of red blood cells.

conditions, the athlete then competes at a normal altitude level and experiences enhanced aerobic endurance. Perhaps you have heard of cities such as Denver or Mexico City where breathing is more difficult, or you may have heard about mountain climbers who have to use oxygen while scaling tall mountains.

When an athlete trains at high altitudes and then competes at lower altitudes, in theory, he or she will have an advantage because the body will be better equipped to process oxygen. While there is undoubtedly some benefit for athletes who train at high altitudes, the effects are not so impressive as to make high-altitude training a major component in preparing for a competition. Those who train at high altitudes may also suffer some dangerous side effects. Among these dangers is

MARCO PANTANI:
THE LONG AND WINDING ROAD

Marco Pantani (Figure 4.2) was more than a preeminent Italian cyclist; he was a national hero. In 1998, Pantani rode his way to victory in both the Tour de France and the Giro (the major Italian cycling race), a pair of feats thought to be nearly impossible. Later, Pantani was accused of using erythropoietin (EPO). Although he never admitted to using EPO, and has never been definitively found to have used EPO through drug testing, the Pantani case raises a fundamental concern: the fact that body enhancing drugs affect all athletes, whether they are actually doping or not.

The test for EPO involves measuring the amount of hemoglobin in the blood. If the hemoglobin level is above 50%, an athlete is considered to be blood doping. During the 1999 Giro race, Pantani was tested and showed a hemoglobin level of 52%. As a result, Pantani felt personally humiliated and became dedicated to establishing his innocence and clearing his name. Since then, his career spiraled down a long and winding path toward his eventual death from unknown causes at the young age of 34 on February 14, 2004.

Source: Rendell, Matt. "The Long, Lonely Road to Oblivion." *The Observer.* March 7, 2004.

hypoxia. This condition occurs when a person does not get enough oxygen. At first, a person who is experiencing hypoxia reacts much like a person who has had a little too much to drink—he or she exhibits poor judgment and experiences a decline in motor coordination. Continued hypoxia, however, is serious and can lead to death.

THE PROBLEM OF TESTING:
ETHICS OF BLOOD DOPING

One thing that differentiates blood doping from other forms of doping is its ability to be detected. In most cases, there are no

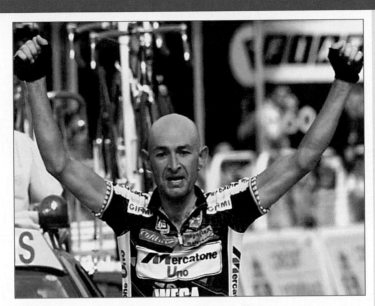

Figure 4.2 *The Italian cyclist Marco Pantani triumphantly crosses the finish line and wins the 15th stage of the 1997 Tour de France. Although Pantani was never officially charged with doping, insinuations of EPO use plagued him throughout his career.*

clear tests to measure blood doping. Any living human being would fail a test for red blood cells, hemoglobin, or EPO. Therefore, alternate tests that compare the proportions of blood cells, hemoglobin, or EPO must be used to detect blood doping. One of the problems with this form of testing is that it is difficult to tell the difference between a person training at high altitude and a person injecting EPO.[7] Naturally, this leads to an ethical problem.

Although techniques of infusion and the use of EPO are clearly outlawed by most athletic organizations, including the Olympics, high-altitude training is not. The main difference

SCIENCE AND TECHNOLOGY

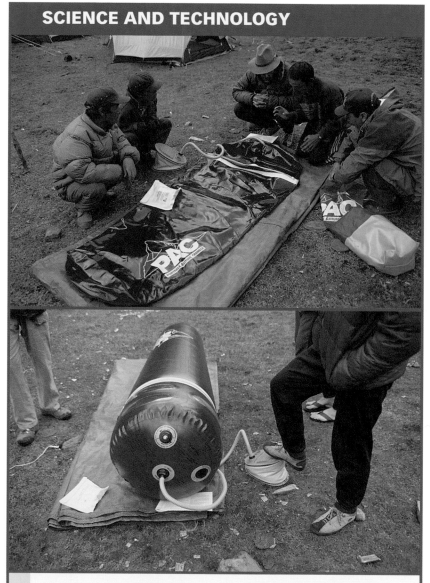

Figure 4.3 *The deflated Gamow Bag (top) is viewed by a number of hikers. It is used at high altitudes where the air is sparse to simulate normal oxygen conditions. The picture on the bottom shows the Gamow Bag inflated and ready to use. Since its inception, the bag has saved numerous lives.*

This bright red, cocoon-shaped bag is called the Gamow® Bag (Figure 4.3). Invented by Dr. Igor Gamow, the Gamow Bag is used at high altitudes (most often by climbers) to simulate sea-level oxygen conditions. The bag effectively treats altitude sickness (hypoxia) and has saved numerous lives. Its predecessor, "the Bubble," did quite the opposite. Gamow was originally working on a chamber that would simulate high-altitude conditions that could be used by athletes to increase hemoglobin levels. Today, many of these portable high-altitude simulation devices are available. They work by removing a portion of the oxygen from the air that circulates inside the chamber. As the athlete sleeps, he or she is able to improve the efficiency with which his or her body captures and uses oxygen.

is that the latter requires real effort. In addition, athletes have argued that autologous blood doping should not be illegal because they are not injecting a "drug"—they are simply using their own blood. With these types of complications, and with no accurate test that can differentiate between forms of blood doping, how can it be controlled? This is a question that has not yet been answered but eventually will have to be, as further biotechnological advances are made, and the line between fair and foul play becomes increasingly difficult to discern.

5

Stimulants, Relaxants, Weight Control, and Pain

Have you ever poured yourself a steaming hot cup of coffee, taken an aspirin for a headache, used cough medicine, or taken a diet pill? These are all examples of drugs used by millions of people to increase energy, relieve pain, or lose weight. These drugs, although widely consumed, can be dangerous at high dosages and can affect an athlete's performance.

Although many people associate steroid use with doping, few understand the wide spectrum of methods and drugs used by athletes. The conventional wisdom of doping is that athletes use drugs to become stronger, but there are many other reasons athletes take performance enhancing drugs. Some athletes use stimulants to quicken their heart rate whereas others use relaxants to slow it down. Some sports, such as boxing and horse racing (sports that have weight requirements) lend themselves well to the use of diuretic drugs, which are used to control weight. Some drugs are not used to create any beneficial effect at all but to take away the pain of an injury so that an athlete can continue to compete while injured.

Although the list of drugs used to stimulate, relax, control weight, and mask pain is extensive, this chapter will focus on the most popular drugs in each class. The classes of doping drugs discussed in this chapter are important for forming a complete understanding of the worldwide doping epidemic.

STIMULANTS

It is no secret that stimulants have been used for thousands of years in one form or another. Stimulants such as cocaine, caffeine, and nicotine have been used in almost all cultures over the course of human history. From South America to the Far East to the United States, these drugs are more popular today than ever before.

For the amateur and professional athlete, stimulants are used for two major reasons: to heighten energy levels and to boost endurance. Athletes have cited many additional effects of stimulants, including increased aggressiveness, the ability to play despite pain, and increased alertness, which provides the opportunity for quicker reactions. Importantly, although scientific studies have unanimously shown the effects of stimulants to include increased heart rate and blood pressure, increased oxygen capacity, stimulated central nervous system, and decreased need for sleep, they are less unified in establishing the level of effect that stimulants have on performance. Some studies have found no correlation between stimulants and increased performance, which has led to their reclassification as placebo drugs (drugs that have no actual physical effect). Still, the fact that stimulant use among athletes is as popular as it is widespread provides good insight into the drug's effects, whether physiological or psychological.

How do Stimulants Work?

There has been considerable debate over how stimulants act on the body. There are many different theories, all of which may be valid in part. In addition, there are many different drugs classified as stimulants, each with its own particular action mechanism and set of effects. It is also known that different people can have dramatically different reactions to the same drug, which makes it difficult to reach uniform conclusions. In the midst of this seemingly confusing situation, there is one commonly accepted explanation for why stimulants work the way they do.

The central nervous system (CNS) is responsible for many bodily activities, including movement and, more importantly for the purposes of this chapter, the release of chemical signals. Within the brain there are more than 100 billion neurons. Neurons, as you may already know, are tiny cells that send signals to each other to coordinate virtually all bodily functions. Each neuron has structures called dendrites and axons (Figure 5.1). Dendrites are long branches that extend from the neuron and bring information into the cell. Axons are long projections from the neuron that send information away. Neurons are separated from each other by a tiny space called a synaptic cleft, or synapse. It is through this space that neurons communicate by sending chemical signals, called neurotransmitters, which in turn stimulate the release of other chemicals (Figure 5.2). It is widely accepted that stimulants such as amphetamine and cocaine encourage neurotransmitters to increase levels of dopamine, a chemical substance that produces a variety of physiological reactions and is related to the production of epinephrine, which creates adrenaline (explaining the stimulating effect).

Amphetamine

Amphetamine is the stimulant most abused by athletes and is also widely used by the general population. Amphetamine is the general term for a large group of stimulant drugs (Table 5.1). Amphetamine is a relatively simple molecule; other stimulants are variations of amphetamine's basic form. Though amphetamine was first used in the 1930s to treat a variety of medical conditions, including narcolepsy, obesity, and depression, amphetamine-containing drugs (also referred to as "amphetamines") were first used for their ergogenic (energy increasing and fatigue reducing) effects during World War II, when they were given to soldiers to keep them alert and aggressive.

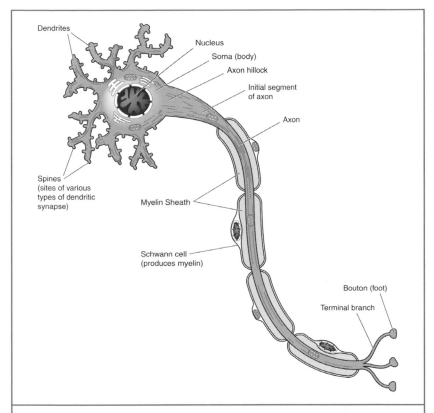

Figure 5.1 **Shown here is a detailed illustration of a nerve cell, or neuron. Your brain has more than 100 billion of these neurons! Neurons are responsible for many bodily activities, including movement and the transmission of chemical signals. Many drugs work by manipulating certain neurotransmitters (the chemicals that send messages between neurons), which in turn have a domino effect, activating one neuron after another to send chemical signals around the body.**

Soon after its entrance onto the battlefield, amphetamine made its first appearance on the playing field. Used by athletes in a host of sports, amphetamine is known to cause an increased heart rate, more rapid metabolism, and decreased fatigue. To the athlete taking part in a strenuous sport that requires great endurance, these effects are clearly seen as positive.

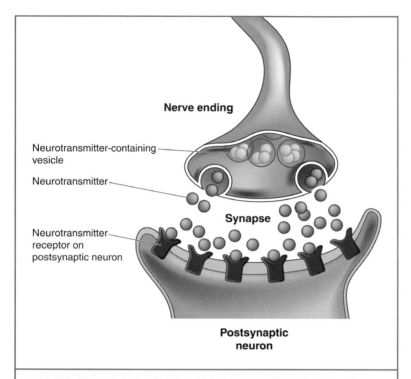

Nerve ending

Neurotransmitter-containing vesicle

Neurotransmitter

Synapse

Neurotransmitter receptor on postsynaptic neuron

Postsynaptic neuron

Figure 5.2 A closer look at the connection between neurons shows how neurotransmitters actually move from neuron to neuron. Here, you can see how neurotransmitters are released from the end of one nerve, move through the synapse, and are collected by receptors on the corresponding nerve. Interestingly, nerve cells adapt over time to the chemicals that are released, which may be part of the reason for long-term drug effects.

Although amphetamine may produce some positive reactions, these effects are clearly outweighed by the problems it causes, which include: insomnia, nervousness, agitation, psychosis, and, at high doses, hyperthermia (overheating) and heart failure. Over the years, amphetamine use has resulted in a number of deaths in athletic competition. Danish cyclist Kurt Enemar Jensen and British cyclist Tommy Simpson died from amphetamine use during the Summer Olympics (1960 and 1967, respectively). Countless other athletes have collapsed in

Table 5.1 Common Amphetamine-Containing Drugs

GENERIC NAME	TRADE NAME	STREET NAME	MEDICAL USE
Racemic amphetamine sulfate	Benzedrine	Bennies, Peaches	Used to treat attention-deficit/ hyperactivity disorder (ADHD)
Dextroamphetamine sulfate	Dexidrine	Dexies, Oranges, Orange hearts	Used to treat attention-deficit/ hyperactivity disorder (ADHD)
Methamphetamine hydrochloride	Desoxyn Methampex	Meth, Crystal, Whites	Used to treat attention-deficit/ hyperactivity disorder (ADHD)
Amphetamine complex	Biphetamine	Black beauties	Used to treat attention-deficit/ hyperactivity disorder (ADHD)

Source: Strauss, Richard H. *Drugs & Performance in Sports*. Philadelphia: W.B. Saunders Company, 1987, p. 70.

competition because of their amphetamine use. As a result, amphetamine is banned by the IOC and is illegal without a written doctor's prescription in most countries. Amphetamine is used legally to treat attention-deficit/hyperactivity disorder (ADHD) and narcolepsy, and to control weight.

Mechanism of Action: Amphetamine

Amphetamine works by manipulating the levels of certain neurotransmitters in the central nervous system (CNS) and the peripheral nervous system (PNS). The CNS is made up of the brain and spinal cord, whereas the PNS includes all the nerves in the rest of the body (including muscle nerves; Figure 5.3). As has already been discussed, the CNS and PNS are made up of billions of nerve cells. When amphetamine is taken, it enters these nerve cells and displaces the

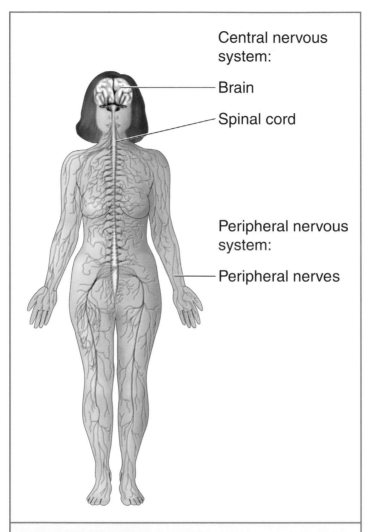

Figure 5.3 The central and peripheral nervous systems consist of the brain, spinal cord, and peripheral nerves that extend to the rest of the body. Drugs such as amphetamine manipulate the release of chemical signals in the brain, which in turn sends signals down the spinal cord and throughout the body. Many drugs such as caffeine and amphetamine do not cause the production or release of additional chemicals but act to block the reabsorption of chemicals, such as dopamine, which results in higher concentrations of these chemicals in the brain.

neurotransmitters noradrenaline and dopamine. Dopamine is a powerful neurotransmitter located and released in the brain, whereas noradrenaline is a primary building block—or precursor—of epinephrine, which increases the heart rate, blood pressure, and the blood sugar level. Normally, these neurotransmitters are released and rapidly recycled by the nerve cells by a process called reuptake. Amphetamine affects the release of these neurotransmitters and also prevents their reuptake. The result is an overabundance of neurotransmitters, which translates into an overly stimulated nervous system in which all bodily systems are operating faster. With continued use, the artificially heightened levels of neurotransmitters result in lower than normal levels after amphetamine cessation, which accounts for many of the adverse effects and the addictive properties of amphetamine.

METHYLPHENIDATE

Methylphenidate, or Ritalin®, as it is more commonly known, is an amphetamine-like prescription given to children with attention-deficit/hyperactivity disorder (ADHD). Interestingly, although methylphenidate acts just like other stimulants in adults, stimulating the central nervous system, it appears to have the opposite effect on children. Ritalin is prescribed for children who are hyperactive, and acts as a calming medication. Doctors are not exactly sure how Ritalin works, but they believe it has to do with stimulating certain neurons in the brain that are not active in children with ADHD. Though the use of this stimulant to treat children has been highly debated, its use in the United States has grown significantly since the early 1990s. The disparate effects that methylphenidate has on children and adults is a good example of how naming the effects of stimulants in a unified manner can be quite difficult.

Caffeine

Caffeine is the most commonly used stimulant in the world, taken not just by athletes but also by a significant portion of the population. Caffeine, like amphetamine, is a drug that stimulates the central nervous system. Caffeine works by binding to adenosine receptors. Adenosine is widely used by the body and is the central component of adenosine triphosphate (ATP), the body's energy storage molecule. Cells secrete adenosine as they lose energy to let the body know that it needs rest. Adenosine is highly linked to sleep. As caffeine binds to adenosine receptors, it blocks the action of adenosine and the body's ability to slow down. With no adenosine around, nerve cells speed up and the brain reacts by releasing adrenaline. Caffeine also works just like other amphetamines to slow down dopamine reuptake.

Caffeine can be found in many products such as coffee, tea, cocoa, soda, chocolate, cough medicine, and diet pills. Because caffeine has ergogenic affects, the IOC has controlled its use by placing limits on the level of caffeine permitted in the bloodstream at the time of competition.

Cocaine

Starting in the 1970s, cocaine use began to supersede the use of amphetamine. This shift took place because the effects of cocaine are similar to those of amphetamine but are significantly heightened. Cocaine, like amphetamine, binds to the dopamine transporter molecule, thereby preventing dopamine from being reabsorbed by the nerve cell. As a result, extra dopamine builds up in the synaptic cleft (the space between two neurons), causing intense feelings of euphoria. Many people use cocaine recreationally for these euphoric effects. Cocaine has many of the same effects and adverse side effects as other stimulants, but at a much stronger level. In addition, cocaine is extremely addictive and can result in a drug habit that easily takes over a person's life. Many athletes have succumbed to cocaine drug abuse and lost their careers as a result.

RELAXANTS

Relaxants, also referred to as depressants, can be placed on the opposite end of the stimulant spectrum. As you would expect, relaxants slow down the central nervous system, causing a series of effects such as drowsiness, impaired judgment, and impaired psychomotor ability. Typically, athletes use relaxants recreationally after competition to calm nerves and "let off steam." Relaxants are used to escape anxiety and, because athletes are particularly susceptible to stressful situations, the

Diego Maradona

Many people believe Diego Maradona was one of the greatest soccer players of all time. Born in Argentina in 1960, Maradona's illustrious career involved stints with Argentinean, Spanish, and Italian teams, leading many to various levels of victory. Maradona brought his native Argentina the World Cup title in 1986. He took Argentina to the World Cup again in 1990 but lost. Though extraordinarily blessed with deft athletic skill, Maradona was also plagued by habitual cocaine abuse. As early as 1990, Maradona's drug use began to affect his game. In 1991, he was banned from soccer after failing a drug test, which showed traces of cocaine. But perhaps the greatest disappointment in his career came in 1994 when he once again brought his team to the World Cup, but was forced to go home in disgrace after again failing a drug test. After retiring from the game in 1997, Maradona has continued to deal with a seemingly insurmountable cocaine addiction. In April 2004, Maradona suffered a heart attack following a cocaine overdose. At the time of this writing, he was receiving drug rehabilitation in Cuba.

use of these drugs among them is persistent. As with stimulants, there are many different drugs that are categorized as relaxants and, likewise, there are many different specific effects and adverse side effects. Relaxants include sedatives, barbiturates, alcohol, marijuana, and beta-blockers. Clinical uses for relaxants include treatment of sleeping disorders, pain relief for patients with severe chronic conditions, and relief of anxiety. Some of the adverse effects include cardiovascular and respiratory depression, withdrawal problems, drowsiness, and decreased psychomotor skills.

WEIGHT CONTROL

Diuretics are another type of body enhancement drug. Athletes competing in sports with weight requirements, such as boxing, horse racing, wrestling, weight lifting, and gymnastics, sometimes use diuretics. Diuretics are also used to pass drug tests because they increase the amount of urine produced by the body. This increase dilutes any drugs in the urine, making them more difficult to identify. Clinically, diuretics are used to regulate blood pressure.

Diuretics work to reduce weight by dehydrating fat cells. Because these cells are 70% water, their dehydration results in temporary weight loss (the cells will eventually rehydrate). This artificial dehydration causes a host of side effects such as cramping, exhaustion, and sometimes cardiac arrest that leads to death.

Although there are various diuretics that work in different ways, diuretics generally work by blocking sodium and water from being absorbed by epithelial cells lining the renal tubule (located in the kidney). This blockage works in various ways, but one of the main mechanisms of action is through the inhibition of protein molecules that are involved in the transfer of electrolytes (*electrolyte* is a scientific word referring to different salts in various bodily fluids). By disabling the protein, these salts are not reabsorbed and are excreted through the urine. The overall result is a lack of water throughout the body, which reduces total weight.

MASKING PAIN

Pain is an unavoidable attribute of competitive sport or any athletic endeavor. Pain is the athlete's archenemy because it can crush athletic performance and cripple the athlete's future. As a result, great pains—so to speak—are taken to combat this unwanted menace. Many of the drugs discussed in this section can and are used to battle the ramifications of pain. When stimulants are taken prior to competition, an athlete may sustain and aggravate an injury without even realizing it. Relaxants and narcotics are also used after a competition to relieve pains sustained during the activity. While pain relievers can serve a legitimate medical function, it is important to understand the danger of using them instead of the body's normal recovery system.

When pain or injury occurs, some part of the body has been stressed beyond its capacity. The body will recover from most injuries in time—but for many athletes, that time is too long. The most important thing for athletes to realize about taking pain relievers is that they are not healing the injury, but merely masking it. The athlete may feel fine, but the broken

"THE SUNDAY SYNDROME"

For a player in the National Football League (NFL), the game means everything. For these modern-day gladiators, pain and injury are just part of the game. Perhaps because of the great physical and mental stress placed upon their shoulders, players in the NFL have been known to abuse amphetamines at an exorbitant level. In a well-publicized study in 1981 called "The Sunday Syndrome: From Kinetics to Altered Consciousness," records dating from 1968 to 1969 showed that an average of 65 amphetamine tablets were taken per player per game among NFL teams (based on purchase records, not official use).

Source: Mandell, A. J., K. D. Stewart, and P. V. Russo. "The Sunday Syndrome: From Kinetics to Altered Consciousness." *Federation Proceedings* 40 (1981): 2693–2968.

bone is still broken, the torn tendon still torn. This creates the potential for exacerbating the injury, making it much worse than it was to begin with.

The paradox of pain relief is highly visible among the world's varying levels of athletes. At the high school and even amateur level, injuries are usually taken very seriously and force a player to sit on the sidelines. At this level, the risk and cost of chronically aggravating the injury is too great to take the chance. At the professional level, however, where playing the game is the athlete's only source of present and future income, athletes will do almost anything to mask pain so that they can keep playing. Ironically, although the job of the physician at amateur levels is ultimately to protect the athlete from long-term damage, the physician treating professional athletes is often forced to leave his or her ethics on the sidelines and provide pain-relieving medications to athletes who run the risk of permanent damage.

6

Nutritional Supplements

Athletes have doped for centuries using many different drugs and methods to increase performance. These drugs and methods constitute a large and varied catalog. Compared to harder and more dangerous forms of performance enhancement drugs, nutritional supplements have significantly fewer dangerous consequences and yield significantly lower ergogenic results. Still, because most athletes engage in nutritional management and supplementation and because there are important distinctions between individual supplements, nutritional supplements are nonetheless a topic in need of attention.

DEFINING NUTRITION

As any athlete knows, nutrition is inseparable from success. A good diet results in a properly functioning body that is able to handle the rigors of athletic competition. For the athlete, nutrition requirements are divided into four phases: training nutrition, pre-competition nutrition, nutrition during competition, and post-competition nutrition. The food pyramid (Figure 6.1) presents a good diet in its most basic form. Maintaining an appropriate and nutritional diet, however, is extremely complicated and there are nutritionists who dedicate entire careers to this scientific study.

There is no single perfect diet. Every athlete—indeed, every person—requires his or her own specific diet to remain healthy. Nutritionists have made general recommendations as to what a

The Food Guide Pyramid

A Guide to Daily Food Choices

KEY
☐ **Fat** (naturally occurring and added)
■ **Sugars** (added)

These symbols show fat and added sugars in foods.

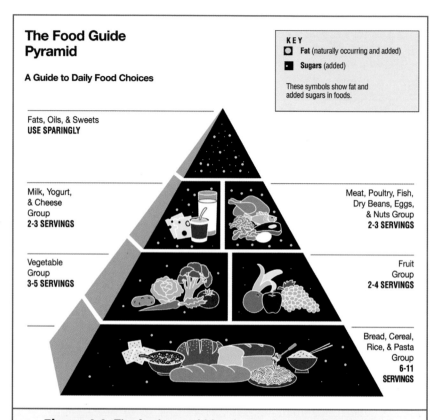

Fats, Oils, & Sweets
USE SPARINGLY

Milk, Yogurt,
& Cheese
Group
2-3 SERVINGS

Meat, Poultry, Fish,
Dry Beans, Eggs,
& Nuts Group
2-3 SERVINGS

Vegetable
Group
3-5 SERVINGS

Fruit
Group
2-4 SERVINGS

Bread, Cereal,
Rice, & Pasta
Group
**6-11
SERVINGS**

Figure 6.1 The food pyramid has been a longstanding model of an appropriate diet. For the average person, a 2,000-calorie diet drawing from all of the groups in the pyramid is the best option to remain healthy, although every individual requires a slightly different diet. Because athletes exert more energy per day than the average person, they often require additional calories to function at full capacity. Interestingly, some diet plans, such as the Atkins® diet, turn the food pyramid upside down, increasing the amount of protein-laden fats while restricting carbohydrates.

good diet includes, as summarized by the food pyramid. Nutrition refers to nourishing the body. Just as there are different grades of fuel for cars, there are different diets for people. An athlete requires the highest-grade fuel in order to compete at his or her best.

DEFINING NUTRITIONAL SUPPLEMENTS

As its name suggests, a nutritional supplement is something added to a regular diet. Sometimes, nutritional supplements are simply added to other foods. Sports drinks, power bars, nutrition or diet shakes, and products with ginseng, echinacea, or other herbal chemicals are all examples of supplements added to a regular diet. Most supplements taken by athletes, however, are vitamin and mineral pills that are taken in addition to food.

The use of nutritional supplements is widespread both within the athletic and general populations. One study, done at the Harvard School of Public Health, found that, in the year 2000, dietary supplement sales reached $15.7 billion, with 48% of Americans indicating that they had used a supplement at one time or another. Reports among athletes have been less consistent, citing supplement use at anywhere between 6 and 96%, depending on the location, type of sport, and scope of the study. More likely, the actual use of nutritional supplements among athletes falls somewhere in the middle of these findings. Whatever the percentage, it is a fact that the use of supplements among athletes and all Americans is drastically increasing from year to year.

Athletes have cited many reasons for using supplements in addition to their normal diets, such as to prevent illness, to increase energy levels, to feel better, to compensate for an inadequate diet, to build muscle, or because of a recommendation from a family member, teammate, nutritionist, or physician. Whether they take the supplements to prevent illness or induce heightened energy levels, athletes should realize that nutritional supplements are completely unregulated in the United States (Figure 6.2). Unlike other drugs prescribed by doctors, nutritional supplements are not subjected to the scrutiny of the Food and Drug Administration (FDA), nor are they tested through clinical trials for safety and efficacy. As a result, the claims made by supplement retailers have not been

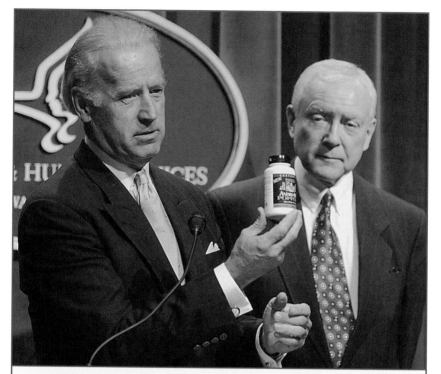

Figure 6.2 Recently, the Food and Drug Administration (FDA) released a warning to consumers concerning the dangers of the nutritional supplement androstendione. Senator Joe Biden of Delaware (left) holds a bottle of Andro Fuel®, which is sold over the counter and advertised as a body enhancement drug. Importantly, drugs classified as nutritional supplements, such as androstendione, are not regulated by the FDA and, therefore, cannot be guaranteed to be safe or effective.

evaluated and the side effects of the products are generally unknown. Only a handful of the most common supplements have been subjected to even minimal scientific examination. Those supplements will be the subject of the rest of this chapter.

Androstenedione

Androstenedione is one of the most popular performance enhancing supplements. Androstenedione is a testosterone precursor and is found naturally in humans, animals, and in some types of plants. When an athlete takes an androstenedione capsule or spray, the chemical is quickly converted into testosterone and estrogen in the body. This reaction takes place in the liver, where an enzyme alters the structure of androstenedione into either estrogen or testosterone. In theory, the effects of this transformation and the subsequent release of testosterone would be the same as those for anabolic androgenic steroids (notice the use of the prefix *andro* in both drugs). Androstenedione acts quickly and its effects last only a short time (1 to 3 hours). Androstenedione is touted by manufacturers to produce the same androgenic results as anabolic steroids without the adverse side effects. Due to the lack of clinical trials and experimentation, however, these claims have not been confirmed.

The few studies that have been conducted on androstenedione have resulted in two alarming conclusions. Studies have found that, while testosterone levels do increase with androstenedione use, estrogen levels increase as well. The cumulative effect of the extra estrogen may cancel out any of the androgenic effect that the testosterone might have. One study, published in the *Journal of the American Medical Association* (*JAMA*), found that androstenedione causes decreased high-density lipoprotein, or HDL, cholesterol levels (the good cholesterol) and increased low-density lipoprotein (LDL) levels (the bad cholesterol). Because there has been little research concerning the side effects of androstenedione, it must be assumed that it has at least some of the same side effects as anabolic androgenic steroids. Androstenedione is currently on the IOC's list of prohibited substances and is banned by the National Football League (NFL) and the National Basketball Association (NBA) as well.

Creatine

Creatine, like androstenedione, is used by athletes to increase strength and is very popular. Creatine is an amino acid that is produced by the liver, kidneys, and pancreas and is also absorbed from foods such as meat and fish.

Creatine is believed to act in the body as an immediate source of energy for muscles by replenishing adenosine triphosphate (ATP) levels. ATP is a molecule that works like a battery, releasing energy when it is needed and storing it when it is not. The amount and level of exercise that a person engages in dictates the amount of creatine and ATP his or her body needs. Creatine is a direct precursor of ATP. In the body, creatine adds a phosphate to adenosine diphosphate (ADP) to create ATP. The ATP is then able to break down again into ADP, a process that releases usable energy. Although creatine exists

ANDROSTENEDIONE AND CREATINE— AMERICA'S PASTIME?

As the smoke cleared from one incredible season, Mark McGwire took his place in the annals of baseball as he broke the single-season home-run record in 1998 by hitting 70 homers. In that magical season, the drama on the field was fueled by the rivalry between Sammy Sosa and McGwire as they battled to become the first to break the outstanding record. Meanwhile, the controversy off the field was McGwire's use of both creatine and andro-stenedione. Through his use of the supplements, and because of the attention his athletic feats received, McGwire became the unwitting poster-child for andro and creatine use. Creatine and androstenedione are not banned by Major League Baseball (MLB). To be fair, McGwire was a home-run hitter long before he started using the supplements and has since stopped using the products, recommending that teenagers stay away from them. Still, the question remains, has America's pastime become andro's heyday?

Source: "Legal in Baseball, McGwire Uses Nutritional Supplement Banned in NFL." CNN Sports Illustrated/Associated Press. August 22, 1998. Available online at *http://sportsillustrated.cnn.com/baseball/mlb/news/1998/08/22/mcgwire_supplement/*.

naturally in the body, supplementation has been linked to increases in short-term muscle strength, though these claims have been disputed. Many researchers say that the drug seems to act as a placebo. The idea is that athletes who take creatine believe they are getting stronger and train harder as a result, creating a self-fulfilling prophecy. Importantly, there is a maximal amount of creatine the body is able to process at any given time. Any more than 20 milligrams of creatine taken in a single day is essentially useless. In addition, it is believed that creatine only works for people who do not have high enough levels to begin with.

Although the side effects of creatine are not fully known, some researchers have noted the possibility of weight gain, nausea, vomiting, diarrhea, and seizures. Currently, creatine is legal in most sports and is completely unmonitored and unregulated.

Chromium

Chromium is an essential trace metal used to reduce weight. Its actual effects, both positive and negative, are not well understood. It is believed that chromium works by assisting cells in glucose uptake. Glucose is the main sugar in the blood and a major source of energy for the body. In theory, the increased sugar extraction efficiency results in a greater use of glucose and, in turn, less storage of glucose in the body's fat reserves. Currently, the exact mechanism through which chromium works to improve glucose uptake are unknown. One theory, however, is that chromium improves insulin receptor ability, leading to the increased glucose efficiency.

Although chromium supplementation is not generally recommended, some scientists believe there is a general chromium deficiency among the American population. Chromium can be obtained from a variety of sources, including meat and even water. Although athletes may have lower levels of chromium as a result of intense exertion, they are more likely to ingest more calories, which compensates for any chromium deficiency they may have.

Ephedra

Ephedra is, or at least was, used by millions of Americans and was widely considered the most dangerous of all supplements used by athletes. Ephedra has been used by athletes and the general population to increase energy and reduce weight. It contains both ephedrine and pseudoephedrine, which are central nervous system stimulants. As a stimulant, ephedra has the same mechanism of action as other amphetamines.

Ephedra has been linked to very serious cardiac side effects with the possibility of death. As such, its use is strongly discouraged. In 2003, the FDA released an alert warning consumers to stop taking ephedra and subsequently banned over-the-counter sales. After intensive study, the FDA found that ephedra "present[ed] an unreasonable risk of illness or injury."

Herbal Products

Over the past decade, there has been an explosion in the use of herbal products such as echinacea, ginseng, and St. John's Wort. A quick look at the vast array of beverages containing

IS EVERYONE TAKING HERBAL PRODUCTS?

Over the past decade, the use of herbal remedies as cures for all kinds of ills has skyrocketed. According to a recent report in the *Washington Post*, 36% of Americans use some form of herbal supplement. Of this 36%, 40% said they used echinacea, 24% said they used ginseng, 21% used ginkgo biloba, and 19% used garlic.

Source: Rob Stein, "Alternative Remedies Gaining Popularity." *Washington Post*. Friday, May 28, 2004, p. A01.

herbal products is a testament to their popularity. There are hundreds, perhaps thousands, of different herbal products on the market and their use is rapidly increasing. As with other nutritional supplements, herbal products have only been minimally studied and cannot be recommended as ergogenic aids. Although various herbal products are touted to have various advantageous health effects, these effects—as well as their adverse effects—are not yet wholly known. In general, however, the side effects and the health benefits of herbal products are not considered to be as bad as those of other body enhancing drugs.

Protein and Amino Acid Supplements

Protein and amino acid supplements are quite common among athletes. Amino acids are the individual molecules that make up protein. There are about 20 amino acids, which string together in chains called peptides that form various protein molecules. A typical protein is made up of more than 500 amino acids linked together. The number and sequence of amino acids determine the protein's function. Some amino acids are made within the body, whereas others, called essential amino acids, must be extracted from food.

Proteins are absolutely necessary for life and affect just about every biological function in the body. Proteins promote growth of muscles, bones, and skin; allow the central nervous system to send impulses; control metabolism; and are the material of which many hormones are made. Although there are seemingly no bad effects of protein and amino acid supplementation, the overabundance of proteins can cause weight gain if not balanced by exercise.

Athletes take protein and amino acid supplements because their use can potentially result in increased growth and functioning of the body. These supplements are not banned by athletic organizations, since they are eaten, through food, daily.

7

Drug Testing: Deception and Detection

With so many body enhancing products and methods available today, the task of accurately and effectively conducting a large-scale drug testing operation can seem like an impossible challenge. Despite the difficulties, scientists are continually developing new ways to detect body enhancing drugs in athletes. The relatively modern inventions of gas chromatography, mass spectrometry, and immunoassays have given hope to sports officials who are charged with the task of cleaning up sports. But adherence to any drug testing policy is a double-edged sword. Drug testing, or doping control, as it is often termed within athletic circles, has always been a reaction-driven science. In other words, as new drugs are created, athletes find new methods to avoid detection, and so new tests must be created in turn. It is a cat-and-mouse chase where, at least in today's world, the testers always seem to be one step behind the dopers.

THE HISTORY OF DRUG TESTING

Although the use of drugs in sports dates back at least to the original Olympic games, testing athletes for drug use is a relatively new endeavor. The first significant steps toward implementing a modern anti-doping policy came in 1960 when the Council of

Europe—an organization of 44 European states established in 1949 as a forum to address human rights issues and other matters of European law—passed a resolution condemning the use of drugs in sports. Following this initial resolution, France became the first nation to adopt a nationwide anti-doping code in 1963. Soon after, in 1965, Belgium and a host of other countries put their own anti-doping codes into effect. Many sports advocates and athletes welcomed the tougher stance against doping, while others were adamantly opposed, but everyone realized that these new codes were essentially, as the classic American proverb goes, "all talk and no action."

The fact that new legislation against doping had little or no impact on actual doping practices in athletics is not to say that the codes were created without good intention. The fundamental difficulty that nations faced in these initial efforts to curb doping in sports was the reality that the technology needed to detect the various doping agents simply did not exist. The situation, however, changed drastically in 1983.

When the first actual athletic drug tests were conducted during the 1968 Olympics in Mexico, the effectiveness and reliability of the testing was viewed with intense skepticism, due chiefly to the lack of sound testing equipment and practices. At this time, athletes were easily able to avoid detection and were therefore not threatened or worried about being caught. In addition, even when drug tests produced results positive for drug use, athletes could argue, with good reason, that the results had been tampered with or were simply wrong.

Much of the confusion surrounding the ability to accurately detect drugs in athletes was eliminated in 1983 when Manfred Donike, a West German professor, first used gas chromatography and mass spectrometry (GC/MS) to detect drug use in sports. The use of these techniques resulted in accurate and consistent testing procedures that dramatically changed the effectiveness of drug testing. Today, thousands of drug tests, conducted by hundreds of athletic organizations around the globe, are done in almost every sport. Problems, however, still remain, as new drugs and methods are created to beat the tests. In addition, many athletes have begun to decry and speak out against aggressive drug testing policies, claiming that drug testing has become a witch-hunt. As with many issues surrounding drug use in sports, there are many differing opinions about drug detection, as well as a host of ethical issues.

DETECTION METHODS

As the variety and complexity of body enhancing products has increased, the methods of detection have evolved in order to keep up. Today, there are highly accurate and scientific machines and techniques that are capable of detecting most enhancement drugs. These systems, however, can only be as accurate as the samples provided to them. Tampering with samples and the altering of results by technicians will always stand in the way of completely valid and reliable testing procedures.

Gas Chromatography

First used for drug testing in 1983, gas chromatography is one of the most common methods of drug detection. The machine on which this test is performed—called a gas chromatograph (Figure 7.1)—is able to analyze both urine and blood samples. The sample is inserted into the machine and vaporized (turned into a gas). The sample then goes through a tube and is broken down into its component parts (metabolites): The different metabolites within the sample vaporize at different times, making it possible to identify them. The time it takes each metabolite to turn into vapor is called its retention time. The time differences are recorded and analyzed by the machine, which is pre-programmed to recognize the retention times of prohibited drugs.

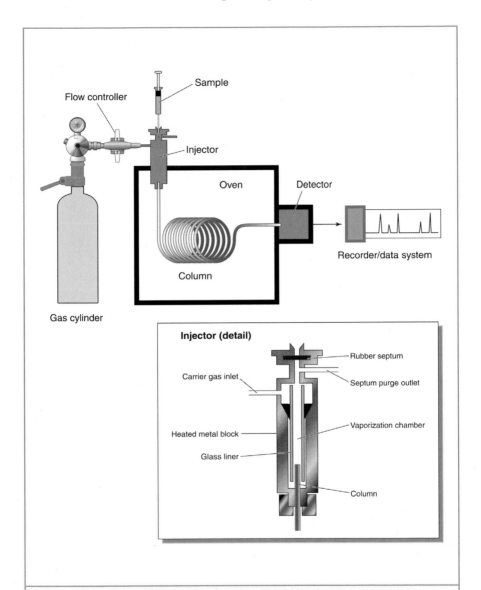

Figure 7.1 Above is a model of the gas chromatography system, which is capable of analyzing both urine and blood. The sample is loaded into the injector and combined with gas, which causes the sample to vaporize. In this gaseous form, the detector is able to identify the various metabolites that make up the sample and determine if any illegal drugs are present.

Mass Spectrometry

Along with gas chromatography, mass spectrometry is one of the most common ways to detect the presence of prohibited drugs. Mass spectrometry is very similar to gas chromatography. The sample is transferred to a gaseous state and then analyzed. The difference is that a mass spectrometer uses an electron beam to separate the sample into its different ions according to their mass. The machine is able to separate all of the ions into groups and measure their concentrations. The metabolites for many enhancement drugs have their own unique structure. The machine is able to analyze the image created by the electron beam and identify specific drugs. Typically, a sample is first run through the gas chromatography phase and, if it is found to contain illicit drugs, it is then run through the mass spectrometer to confirm the initial results.

Immunoassays

Immunoassays are another way to detect foreign substances in urine samples. Immunoassays detect antibodies, which are proteins produced by the body as part of the immune response that can recognize and bind to a specific substance. To test for illegal body enhancing drugs, scientists find antibodies for the metabolite traces left by drugs in the urine. The urine and a solvent that contains the antibodies are mixed together. Scientists are then able to tell whether a drug is present by the reaction between the two substances. Immunochemical assays are very common in all kinds of scientific research. Generally, however, immunoassays are less desirable than GC/MS analyses. Although immunoassays are cheaper and quicker to perform, they sometimes result in false positives. For this reason, GC/MS is the preferred method of detection.

SUBSTANCES USED TO MASK DRUG USE

One of the problems facing drug testers is the fact that there are many drugs and methods athletes can use to avoid drug detection. Drug tests can utilize hair, saliva, and blood samples, but urine is the most common source through which drugs are detected. When a person takes a drug, it is broken down into various components. These components are then absorbed into different areas of the body. Some parts of all drugs are inevitably extracted by the liver and kidneys and released as urine. The components of the drug that end up in the urine are called metabolites. Both dopers and testers are concerned with these metabolites for very different reasons. Dopers use drugs or methods that hide, or "mask," metabolites, whereas testers examine the metabolites in urine to detect various drugs. The most common masking drugs as well as the most common detection methods will be discussed in this section.

Epitestosterone

Epitestosterone is a naturally occurring hormone in the body that is analogous to testosterone. When taken on its own, epitestosterone has no performance enhancing qualities. It also has no serious adverse side effects. Athletes take epitestosterone not for the intrinsic qualities of the hormone itself, but in order to hide the use of testosterone, which *does* have androgenic effects. Typically, the test for anabolic androgenic steroids and the detection of illegal testosterone use involves calculating the testosterone/epitestosterone ratio (T/E ratio). In the average human, the ratio of testosterone to epitestosterone is one to one. According to the IOC, if an athlete's T/E tests above 6:1, then he or she is considered to be using testosterone. By taking epitestosterone, an athlete is able to manipulate the T/E ratio, balancing out the amounts of testosterone and epitestosterone in the body and avoiding detection.

Secretion Inhibitors

Most foods contain substances called organic acids. Many of the drugs athletes use have properties that are similar in structure to these organic acids. The body, specifically the kidneys, has a protein whose function is to remove acids from substances that enter the body and transport them into the urine to be excreted. Secretion inhibitors act as protein blockers, essentially keeping the protein responsible for acid removal from doing its job. If the protein is disabled, the organic acids are not removed and will therefore not show up on a drug test. Clinically, secretion inhibitors are used to treat gout, a condition involving an overabundance of uric acid in the body. Secretion inhibitors, by blocking organic acids from getting into the urine, can disrupt drug tests. Side effects of secretion inhibitors include allergic reactions, kidney problems, vomiting, and nausea.

Diuretics

As previously discussed, drug tests work by measuring and identifying metabolites in urine. Some athletes, in order to avoid detection, use diuretics. Diuretics allow an athlete to reduce his or her weight because they extract water from cells throughout the body (see Chapter 5). The water that is extracted causes an increase in urine flow, which, in turn, dilutes the amount of drug metabolites in the urine and makes them harder to detect.

Plasma Expanders

Plasma expanders work by increasing the fluid component of blood. They are often used by emergency medical responders to stabilize victims who have experienced massive blood loss. When a person loses too much blood, he or she is susceptible to shock and, if blood loss continues, death can result. Plasma expanders act as artificial blood by increasing the total volume of blood in the body. Plasma expanders have no significant side effects, except the possibility of allergic reactions. They can also be used as masking drugs, because they dilute the concentration of illegal substances in the blood, making them harder to detect. Specifically, some athletes use plasma expanders to hide the use of erythropoietin (EPO).

Additional Methods of Avoiding Detection

While some athletes use drugs to mask other drugs, the most common methods used by athletes do not involve the use of any natural or artificial substances at all. One method athletes use to avoid detection involves urine switching. That is, before an athlete is tested, he or she gets a sample of someone else's urine and uses it to pass the drug test. This method, though effective, has become rare and more difficult as testing agencies now frequently require the athlete to produce the sample at the testing site.

Perhaps the most common method of avoiding detection as well as the biggest problem testers face is the use of time. All drugs have what is called a "period of detectability." This means that all drugs are broken down, used, and discarded by the body in a certain amount of time, called the drug clearance time. If an athlete knows how much time it takes for a certain drug to leave the body and knows when he or she will be tested, simple math will allow the athlete to avoid detection. The situation is complicated, however, by the fact that different drugs have different clearance times. Anabolic androgenic steroids, for example, have much longer clearance times than stimulants. The most effective way to deter this practice is the use of random testing, in which the athlete has no idea when a drug test might take place.

CURRENT PROBLEMS AND ETHICAL ISSUES

As drug detection technology continues to improve and scientists are better able to accurately test large groups of athletes, the ethical issues of drug testing increase as well. One major problem facing testers is the use of new enhancing drugs that cannot be detected. Today, there are no completely accurate tests for many drugs such as human growth hormone and

EPO. Illegal use of these substances cannot be detected because they are found naturally in the body. If a test to detect their presence were used, no human being could pass. Although there are tests being developed for these enhancement products, the creation of more undetectable drugs to take their place can be expected.

Another problem facing today's sporting organizations, if they wish to eradicate or control drug use, is the disparity between the resources for testers and the resources for dopers. Doping is a big business with millions of dollars at stake. Although many of the drugs can be obtained legally over the counter or from other countries without restrictions, there are many others that must be obtained by illegal means. Much like the drug dealer selling cocaine or heroin, the dealer selling doping products, often called a "guru," works in a high-risk, high-reward business. Even though gurus can expect serious legal consequences and jail time if caught selling illegal substances, the money athletes are willing to pay for their services seems to justify the risk for many gurus. As long as there is more money invested on the guru side of the doping game than on the tester side, the gurus will inevitably have the advantage.

While new drugs and a lack of funds will probably always haunt their work, drug testers are also continually stalked by the ethical implications of their work. One ethical dilemma related to drug testing is the occurrence of mistakes. Many athletes feel that because of the possibility of testing mistakes, which could result in unfair suspensions, testing should not be used. This argument, however, is increasingly hard to make as the drug testing process becomes more accurate. Another issue arises from the extreme complexity of doping control and the number of prohibited substances. Many of the substances prohibited by athletic organizations can be found in clinically useful and common medications. This means that many athletes will test positive for drugs that are being used to treat health problems and not to enhance performance. In addition, testers are often criticized for concentrating so heavily on the use of doping agents that they are ruining sports. Clean athletes will often complain that the attention given to the doper stains the sport and hurts the reputation of all participants. Whether you personally side with the arguments of the dopers or the testers, one thing is clear: Both will continue to jostle for victory in the doping game of the future.

8

Teenage Trends and Attitudes

A common misconception about body enhancing drugs is that only Olympic and professional athletes use them. Many people believe that only these high-level athletes, who earn tremendous amounts of money and are under extreme pressure to succeed, have enough incentive to take harmful and illegal substances to boost perform-ance. Many also think that only these athletes—who have daily access to physicians, personal trainers, and nutritionists—would, in turn, have access to illicit drugs (as well as nutritional supplements such as creatine and androstendione).

On the topic of performance enhancing drugs, conventional wisdom is not correct. In truth, teenage athletes, and, in fact, any teenager is just as likely to be taking body enhancing drugs as an elite athlete. Many performance enhancing agents—particularly nutritional supplements such as creatine and androstendione—are easily available to anyone. Historically, professional athletes and teens make up the vast majority of body enhancement drug users. Some of the reasons teenagers use these substances are the same as those for high-level athletes: pressure to succeed, emphasis on winning at all costs, and a "bigger is better" attitude. These concepts are not restricted only to high-level sports. High school athletes often feel the same pressure to win, the same yearning for victory, and the same desire to be the best that people like Barry Bonds and Mark McGwire feel.

Teenagers, however, are bombarded by additional pressures that compound and expand their susceptibility to enhancement drug abuse. It is no secret that the urge to "fit in" and be "sexy" are strong incentives to all teenagers to use dangerous products to feel more comfortable with their peers. But how many teenagers today are actually using body enhancing drugs? Why do they use them and where and how do they get them? Finally, what are the health implications that make these drugs specifically harmful to teens? Because it is important for all teenagers, not just athletes, to understand body enhancement drug abuse, these topics will be explored in this section.

TRENDS IN TEENAGE PERFORMANCE ENHANCEMENT DRUG USE

Overall, from 2002 to 2003, there was a slight decline in the use of body enhancement drugs by teenagers. Specifically, the use of amphetamines and stimulants decreased among all adolescents, whereas steroid use only decreased among 10th graders. The following are current data for the use of various body enhancing drugs according to the 2003 Monitoring the Future Study (MTF) and research by the well-known Mayo Clinic:

- 8.4% of 8th graders, 13.1% of 10th graders, and 14.4% of 12th graders were found to be using amphetamines. From 2002–2003, overall use fell at each grade level by 0.4, 1.8, and 2.4% respectively.

- The use of sedatives by 12th graders in 2003 was 8.8%, representing a 0.7% drop from the previous year.

- The use of alcohol among teens remained stable for 8th, 10th, and 12th graders, at 45.6%, 66%, and 76.6% respectively.

- The use of steroids was found to be 2.5% for 8th graders, 3.0% for 10th graders and 3.5% for 12th graders. While steroid use went down overall from 2002 to 2003, it only fell by an average of 0.5%.

- According to a 1999 study conducted by the Mayo Clinic, the percentage of teens using creatine was 8.2%.

WHY DO TEENS USE BODY ENHANCING DRUGS?

With so much information available about the negative effects of body enhancing drugs, and with data suggesting that teenagers do perceive enhancement drugs in a negative light, why is enhancement use on the rise? Here are some possible explanations:

- The high school athlete, like any athlete, will inevitably reach a plateau in performance and may turn to drugs to get past this barrier.

- Teenagers may be curious about enhancing products without recognizing the adverse effects.

- In most schools, drugs tests are not concentrated on performance enhancing drugs, so there is little risk of being caught.

- Performance enhancers are easy to acquire, some being sold over the counter.

- Teens recognize that professional athletes use enhancement drugs and may be encouraged to follow suit.

- Parents and coaches may not actively dissuade teenagers from using performance enhancement drugs.

- Teens may take body enhancement drugs as a reaction to peer and societal pressures that hold up lean, muscular bodies as the ideal.

Although the results from other studies are slightly higher or slightly lower than those reported here, the MTF study is conducted by the National Institute on Drug Abuse and is a reputable source for drug use statistics. Though some people might think the percentages of teen body enhancement drug are rather small (they are, in fact, lower than the percentages for the use of other illegal drugs, such as marijuana), they still represent a level that poses a threat to a significant number of America's youth.

It is generally accepted that the number of teens using body enhancement drugs is larger than the number indicated by any study. There are several reasons for this. For example, respondents may give false answers and school testing procedures are sometimes faulty.

Testing for body enhancement drugs in school is a controversial and difficult issue. In addition to the usual arguments concerning the invasion of privacy that occur at every social level and within all athletic organizations, schools have the additional problem of finding the funds needed to implement an effective drug testing program. The price of drug tests varies according to the drug being tested, but generally a single test costs between $10 and $30. Schools, which already operate on extremely tight budgets, are often unwilling or unable to try to obtain the money for drug testing programs. Because money dedicated to drug testing would invariably take money away from other school programs, parents are often hesitant to lobby schools for stricter testing policies. In addition, many parents do not fully recognize the level of risk that body enhancement drugs pose.

Perhaps because of cash constraints or simply because they are trying to be efficient, schools that do implement testing programs often test only athletes for drug use. Although there are arguments both for and against the policy of targeting only athletes, the fact remains that statistics generally do not reflect drug use among entire school populations.

Anabolic Steroid Use Among Teens

The use of steroids among teens, while decreasing slightly from 2002 to 2003, has generally increased over the last decade (Figure 8.1). In 2003, 3.5% of 12th graders admitted using steroids, an increase of 1.4% from 1991. Furthermore, based on a collection of data in 1995, approximately 375,000 adolescent males and 175,000 females had used anabolic steroids at least once. To date, all studies have found that more male adolescents use steroids than females, but this may change in the future.

One of the more alarming statistics regarding adolescent steroid use is the rise in prevalence among teenage girls. The Monitoring The Future (MTF) study found that the percentage of females using steroids increased by 100% between 1991 and 1996. This trend has continued and shows no signs

WHERE DO TEENS GET BODY ENHANCING DRUGS?

Although many people believe that only high-level professional athletes have access to body enhancing drugs, the reality is that the drugs are much easier to obtain than most people imagine. A simple Internet search can provide a host of enhancement drug outlets. Here are a few ways through which teenagers might acquire performance drugs:

- Local nutrition stores that sell legal body enhancing products.
- Dealers at school or on the streets who sell enhancers in addition to all kinds of other drugs.
- Parents' medicine cabinets that are stocked with prescription drugs.
- Friends who have legitimate prescriptions.
- The Internet.

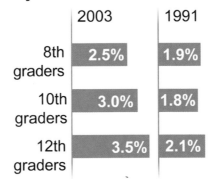

High school steroid use is on the rise

More teenagers are using steroids, according to a national survey of 50,000 high school students conducted at the University of Michigan's Institute for Social Research.

Percentage of students who said they had used steroids

	2003	1991
8th graders	2.5%	1.9%
10th graders	3.0%	1.8%
12th graders	3.5%	2.1%

SOURCE: University of Michigan   AP

Figure 8.1 Over the last decade, the number of teenagers using steroids has increased. A study conducted at the University of Michigan found that 3.5% of high school seniors used anabolic androgenic steroids.

of slowing down soon. These figures are particularly frightening because many of the negative effects of steroids on females are irreversible.

Although steroid use is generally increasing among adolescents, one positive finding is that the perception of steroids as harmful drugs is on the rise as well. The 1998 MTF study found that 68.1% of 12th graders believed steroids were a great risk and 91.4% of 12th graders disapproved of steroid use. Though teenagers may increasingly see steroids as harmful drugs, 44.5% nonetheless said that it would be easy for them to get steroids.

TEENAGE ENHANCEMENT DRUG USE AND IMAGE

This book has concentrated heavily on the way that enhancement drugs are used by athletes and in sport. For many teens, however, the use of enhancement drugs has little or nothing to do with athletics but rather with appearance. The pressure for teenagers to look good (or "hot"), in addition to a host of other social pressures surrounding drug use, is well documented. For teens, there are two overriding reasons that lead to the use of enhancement drugs: the pressure to be thin and the pressure to be muscular.

In today's world, so called "miracle programs" like the South Beach Diet® and the Atkins Diet are extremely popular. Less well known is the fact that many teenagers, both boys and girls, go beyond typical dieting to lose weight—resorting to a host of dietary supplements. According to a 1993 study of more than 11,000 high school students conducted by the Centers for Disease Control and Prevention (CDC), over 33% of girls and 15% of boys considered themselves overweight. According to the National Center for Disease Statistics, during the same time period, 11% of adolescent girls and boys were *actually* overweight (today that figure is 16%).The increase in the perception of being overweight has translated into an increase in the number of teenagers using diet pills.

Most diet pills include forms of ephedrine among their ingredients. Caffeine and chromium are also common drugs used to speed up metabolism and lose weight. What is important for teens to know about these drugs is that they do have adverse effects and that they only represent a "quick fix." Although taking diet pills may cause short-term weight loss, only a balanced, nutritious diet, combined with exercise, can result in long-term weight reduction.

In addition to losing weight, many teens are concerned with developing lean, muscular physiques. As a result, the use of anabolic steroids among teens has generally increased over the last decade. Although anabolic steroids do, in fact, increase muscle mass, as discussed in Chapter 3, the adverse effects may far outweigh any potential gains in muscle. Additionally, experts have concluded that steroids only have a significant effect when coupled with the extensive physical training undertaken by athletes. Whether the drugs are used to improve athletic performance, or simply to improve appearance, there are specific health implications that make teenage use particularly risky.

SPECIFIC HEALTH IMPLICATIONS

Although the use of performance enhancing drugs is not encouraged for any group of people, teenagers who use enhancers are at particular risk of experiencing dangerous side effects. Many people mistakenly believe enhancement drugs make you healthier. To be clear, these drugs may make you temporarily stronger, faster, or more energetic, but they will *not* make you healthier. In the long run, the negative effects of most body enhancing drugs far outweigh any short-term benefits.

The main reason enhancement drugs are even more dangerous for teens than for adults is that teenagers are still growing. In order for the body to grow properly, teenagers need a good diet and plenty of exercise. The use of dietary pills, stimulants, steroids, and other performance enhancers disrupts the body's natural growth process. It is known, for example, that steroids are particularly dangerous for teens because they send an early signal to the brain to stop producing testosterone, which results in stunted growth.

There is an additional risk that teens run because they are often poorly informed about enhancement drugs to begin with. Professional athletes who use these drugs usually have trainers and doctors who monitor their health. These medical experts know how to use the drugs to produce the fewest possible problems. They also know the quantity and route by which enhancers will cause the fewest side effects. Teens, for the most part, do not have access to medical experts and are therefore susceptible to extreme errors. Teens often end up taking such high quantities of these drugs that their enhancing effects are completely outweighed by their unhealthy side effects.

Clearly, body enhancing drugs pose significant risks to teenagers. To make matters worse, teenagers often see themselves as invincible and are either unaware or unwilling to admit that these drugs have harmful effects. Current trends project that the use of body enhancing drugs will continue

BEYOND SPORT: BOTOX® AND BEAUTY

As Americans become increasingly conscious of their appearance, new methods are utilized and greater lengths are taken to obtain beauty. Today, a product called Botox is one of the most popular medications used for this purpose. As an enhancer, Botox is used to get rid of wrinkles. Botox is the neurotoxin, botulinum toxin A, a chemical similar to the poison that causes botulism (a type of food poisoning). Botox works by blocking proteins that normally allow nerves to fire and muscles to contract. Essentially, Botox freezes the muscle so that it is unable to move; hence, no wrinkle can form. However, Botox does not prevent wrinkles—it only hides them.

to rise among teens in the future. As a result, increased drug testing and stricter regulations can be expected. Because it is important for people to understand the legal consequences of body enhancement drug use, it is that topic we will discuss in the next chapter.

9

Enhancement, Ethics, and the Law

We know that body enhancing drugs have adverse side effects, many of which have been discussed, but indulging in enhancement invites legal trouble as well. The laws and regulations surrounding body enhancers are as complex and numerous as the number of drugs that are available. The laws also provide for a wide range of punishments—from suspension from sports to jail time. The variety of legal actions taken against people who take enhancers are both interesting and important—interesting because they raise many ethical concerns dealing with personal freedom, and important because athletes and others using enhancing drugs must realize that many of these drugs carry severe legal consequences that can destroy careers and ruin reputations.

THE HISTORY OF DRUG CONTROL

Unlike the history of body enhancement drug abuse, the history of drug control is comparatively short. In the United States, drug control dates back to the 1840s, when Congress passed the National Drug Import Law to ensure that imported drugs were properly labeled. Before this time, drugs were totally unregulated by the U.S. government and, moreover, there were no established definitions for prescription and nonprescription drugs, narcotics, or drug abuse. Furthermore, there were no laws requiring manufacturers of drugs to report the quantity and distribution of drugs produced, to conduct tests to make sure that drugs were safe, or to carry out clinical trials to prove that a drug worked. In fact, until the 1906 Food and Drug Act was passed, anyone could make or take a concoction or sell any drug to anyone they wanted without fear of any legal repercussions. The world we live in today, however, is very different. Drug policies, agencies, and laws have vastly grown and evolved. Here are a few of the highlights:

- **1906 Pure Food and Drug Act:** Arguably the most important piece of food and drug legislation in American history, the 1906 act defined both *drug*[8] and *misbranding* (falsely labeling a food or drug product so that it is not what the label says it is)[9] and was designed to eliminate false claims. The act directly led to the creation of the Food and Drug Administration (FDA).

- **1912 Shirley Amendment:** Soon after the 1906 Act, the government realized that there were innumerable violations that needed attention. In essence, the 1906 act only prohibited false claims about the ingredients of a product—not its intended purpose. The Shirley Amendment was the first attempt by the government to remove fraudulent drugs (drugs that did not do what they claimed to do) from the market.

- **1938 Food, Drug, and Cosmetic Act:** This act required drug manufacturers to document and prove the safety of all their drugs and report their findings to the FDA.

- **1951 Durham Humphrey Act:** This act made a distinction, for the first time, between prescription and nonprescription drugs. As a result, many medications can now only be obtained with a physician's prescription.

- **1962 Kefauver-Harris Amendment:** This legislation dealt with the effectiveness of new drugs. As a result, manufacturers now had to prove that their drugs were not only safe but also effective.

- **1970 Controlled Substance Act:** This important piece of legislation outlines the control, evaluation, and penalties of all narcotic agents and other dangerous drugs. As a result of this act, drugs are now classified into five "schedules," according to their medical uses and potential addictive properties (Table 9.1).

- **1990 Steroid Trafficking Act:** This act effectively added steroids to the list of controlled substances as Schedule III drugs, placing their possession and illegal distribution on par with cocaine and other dangerous drugs.

LEGAL CONSEQUENCES OF ENHANCEMENT ABUSE

The legal ramifications of using performance enhancement drugs are extremely diverse. Rules, regulations, prohibited substance lists, and penalties depend on many factors. Each enhancer, for example, has its own set of penalties; each sport has its own list of prohibited substances; each state is free to make its own drug laws; and all penalties depend on the individual situation (having a larger quantity of a drug, for instance, will result in a bigger penalty). Overriding these major differences is the federal list of controlled substances that are mandated by the Drug Enforcement Administration (DEA).

One of the major problems with attempting to control the use and trafficking of enhancement drugs is that most drugs have legitimate medical uses and are manufactured legally by many different pharmaceutical companies. This means that, unlike cocaine or heroin, most enhancement drugs are legal if a person has a prescription from a physician. Furthermore, of the drugs that are controlled in the United States, such as anabolic androgenic steroids, many are not regulated in the rest of the world. As a result, obtaining enhancement drugs can be very easy.

Another concern is that enhancement is not always a "drug" but can be a method as well. Blood doping by reinjecting

Table 9.1 Scheduling of Selected Enhancement Drugs

SCHEDULE	POTENTIAL FOR ABUSE	MEDICAL USE	EXAMPLES	COMMON MAXIMUM PENALTIES FOR TRAFFICKING*
I	High	None	Heroin, Marijuana, THC	**FIRST OFFENSE:** Between 10 years and life in prison; Between $1 million and $4 million fine
				SECOND OFFENSE: Between 20 years and life in prison; Between $2 million and $8 million fine
				2 OR MORE PRIOR OFFENSES: Life imprisonment
II	High	Yes	Amphetamine, Cocaine	Same as Schedule I
III	Less than I and II	Yes	Ephedrine capsules, Anabolic steroids, Barbiturates, Methandros-tenolone (Dianobol), Nandrolone (Deca-Durabolin), Testosterone	**FIRST OFFENSE:** 5 years in prison; $250,000 fine
				SECOND OFFENSE: 10 years in prison; $500,000 fine
IV	Low	Yes	NA	NA
V	Lower than IV	Yes	NA	NA

* These penalties represent the maximum possible trafficking punishments for most drugs in each respective schedule. Trafficking refers to the intent to distribute; penalties are generally less in possession cases. Many drugs, such as cocaine, heroin, and marijuana have their own specific penalties. Penalties vary in relation to the quantity of drug involved.

Source: Drug Enforcement Administration. Available online at *http://www.usdoj.gov/dea/agency/penalties.htm*.

one's own blood, for example, does not require the use of any drug. Therefore, while this method is prohibited by most athletic organizations, it is technically not a criminal offense. There is a clear separation between criminal offenses and athletic offenses. Many enhancement drugs are prohibited in sports but not in the rest of society. Take caffeine, for example. There are no penalties for owning or selling coffee, but for an athlete, too much caffeine could result in disqualification from competition. If this example represents one side of the enhancement law spectrum, anabolic androgenic steroids represent the other.

THE RECLASSIFICATION OF ANABOLIC ANDROGENIC STEROIDS AS A SCHEDULE III CONTROLLED SUBSTANCE

After the initial use of anabolic androgenic steroids (AAS) by the German Army during World War II, the drugs' infiltration into the general population steadily increased. In the United States during the 1980s, a collection of nationwide studies brought attention to the growing problem of steroid abuse, most alarmingly among the adolescent population. One government study, undertaken in 1989, found that 6% of high school males were using steroids.

As a result of the increasing steroid problem, the government responded by enacting the Steroid Trafficking Act of 1990. At the heart of this act was the placement of the 27 most popular and harmful AAS on the Controlled Substance List. As a result of the act, these steroids were listed as Schedule III drugs under federal control. This meant that all manufacturers of AAS would have to register with the DEA, which could then monitor the distribution of AAS throughout the country.

In addition, the law drastically increased the penalties for possessing and distributing steroids illegally. Currently, a first offense of illegal steroid possession in any amount can result in a maximum 5-year prison sentence or a $250,000 fine. For a second offense, the penalty increases to a maximum 10-year prison term or a $500,000 fine.[10] Generally, the 1990 act is considered to have been successful in curbing the domestic diversion of AAS from manufacturers to illegal distributors. Still, the DEA recognizes that many illegal operations exist both at home and abroad, making AAS a persistent problem.

As recently as 2004, President George W. Bush brought national attention to the steroid problem in his State of the Union Address:

> To help children make the right choices, they need good examples. Athletics play such an important role in our society, but, unfortunately, some in professional sports are not setting much of an example. The use of perform-ance-enhancing drugs like steroids in baseball, football, and other sports is dangerous, and it sends the wrong message—that there are shortcuts to accomplishment, and that performance is more important than character. So tonight I call on team owners, union representatives, coaches, and players to take the lead, to send the right signal, to get tough, and to get rid of steroids now.

Clearly, the problem of performance enhancement will continue to pervade not just the athletic community but our society as a whole. And just as the proponents of enhancement control will continue to cajole legislators, so too will those who seek to keep enhancement drugs available navigate the murky waters of new and tougher laws.

ETHICAL CONCERNS

The problem with establishing certain agents as body enhancement drugs and the difficulties that governing bodies have had in enacting regulation are clear roadblocks to the advancement of fair athletic competition. Once enhancement drugs are defined, there are other ethical problems to be considered, dealing primarily with the conflict between freedom and paternalism.

Paternalism, derived from the Latin root *pater*, meaning "father," refers in this case to the limitation of freedom by a regulating body. As when a parent sets a child's curfew, there may be a difficult and heated debate over what is fair and unfair. There are always multiple and usually opposing perspectives involved in the debate. Consider a father who tells his daughter that she must be home by 11:00 P.M. You can imagine the daughter quickly interjecting, "But Dad, everyone else is allowed out until midnight!" The argument over whether body

IN THE REAL WORLD: THE BALCO DEBACLE—WISDOM OR WITCH-HUNT?

In the weeks leading up to the 2004 Summer Olympic Games in Athens, Greece, several top U.S. athletes came under fire for supposed enhancement violations. At the center of the controversy was the Bay Area Laboratory Cooperative (BALCO), a health facility that provides legal supplements and drug testing to professional and Olympic athletes. BALCO was accused of illegally distributing undetectable steroids to high-level athletes. Although indictments have already been handed down to BALCO's founder and vice president as well as to certain high-level athletes, the controversy continues. Additional athletes have been accused of doping, even though they never tested positive. The U.S. Anti-Doping Agency is now asking for athletes to be taken out of competition for what they call "non-analytical positives." This means that athletes can be accused of doping just because they have been associated with BALCO. While the accusations may or may not be valid, some have raised the question: Is it fair to accuse athletes of doping violations without positive drug tests? Does doing so create the risk of treating someone as guilty until proven innocent, of creating a witch-hunt?

enhancing drugs should be used in sport is similar. Is it fair to ban a drug in one sport, but not all sports? If a drug is illegal in one country but not in another, how can there be fair play internationally? Is a drug ban that is implemented but not properly enforced unfair to athletes who observe the ban but then have to compete against athletes who do not? These are tough questions that are consistently and hotly debated. Most governments and athletic organizations have agreed that banning certain drugs is essential for maintaining the integrity of sports and for establishing a fair environment in which athletes can compete. But there are drugs used today for which no reliable tests are available, and with so many natural and legal enhancing supplements around, the line between what is a drug and what is not is becoming increasingly hard to draw. In the future, governments, athletic organizations, athletes, spectators, and all members of society will continue to deal with and debate these issues, and although the arguments are by no means simplistic or one-sided, the future of sporting will depend on their answers.

Notes

1 The reader should know that throughout this text, the terms, *body enhancement* and *performance enhancement* are used interchangeably as they are used throughout the literature.

2 Drape, Joe. "McGwire Admits Taking Controversial Substance." *New York Times.* August 22, 1998.

3 Wadler, Gary I. *Doping in Sport: From Strychnine to Genetic Enhancement, It's A Moving Target.* Available online at *http://www.law.duke.edu/sportscenter/wadler.pdf.*

4 Hemingway, Ernest. *The Old Man and the Sea.* New York: Scribner, p. 103.

5 Nova Online: Amazing Heart Facts. Public Broadcasting Service. Available online at *http://www.pbs.org/wgbh/nova/heart/heartfacts.html.*

6 USA Today. Available online at *http://www.usatoday.com/sports/cycling/2004-07-25-tour-notes_x.htm.*

7 Currently, a test for EPO does exist; however, an ethical argument still remains.

8 The act defines *drug* as "all medicines and preparations recognized in the United States Pharmacopoeia or National Formulary for internal or external use, and any substance or mixture of substances intended to be used for the cure, mitigation, or prevention of disease of either man or other animals."

9 The act declares: "that the term, 'misbranded,' as used herein, shall apply to all drugs, or articles of food, or articles which enter into the composition of food, the package or label of which shall bear any statement, design, or device regarding such article, or the ingredients or substances contained therein which shall be false or misleading in any particular, and to any food or drug product which is falsely branded as to the State, Territory, or country in which it is manufactured or produced."

10 U.S. Drug Enforcement Administration. "Title 21—Food And Drugs, Chapter 13—Drug Abuse Prevention And Control, Subchapter I—Control And Enforcement. Part D—Offenses and Penalties." *Controlled Substances Act.* Available online at *http://www.usdoj.gov/dea/pubs/csa/841.htm#b.*

Bibliography

Books:

Stark, Richard W., Marion Fournier, Jean-Michel Johnson, Gilles Chiasson, eds. *The Drug File: A Comprehensive Bibliography on Drugs and Doping in Sport.* Gloucester, Ontario: Sports Information Resource Centre, 1991.

Strauss, Richard H. *Drugs & Performance in Sports.* Philadelphia: W.B. Saunders Company, 1987.

Taylor, William N. *Anabolic Steroids and the Athlete.* Jefferson, NC: McFarland and Company, Inc., 1982.

———. *Macho Medicine—A History of the Anabolic Steroid Epidemic.* Jefferson, NC: McFarland and Company, Inc., 1991.

Thomas, John A., ed. *Drugs, Athletes, and Physical Performance.* New York: Plenum Medical Book Co., 1998.

Tricker, Ray, and David C. Cook. *Athletes at Risk: Drugs and Sport.* Dubuque, IA: Wm. C. Brown Publishers, 1990.

Voy, Robert. *Drugs, Sport, and Politics.* Champaign, IL: Leisure Press, 1991.

Williams, Melvin H. ed. *Ergogenic Aids in Sport.* Champaign, IL: Human Kinetics Publishers, Inc., 1983.

Wilson, Wayne, and Edward Derse, eds. *Doping in Elite Sport: The Politics of Drugs in the Olympic Movement.* Champaign, IL: Human Kinetics Publishers, Inc., 2001.

Yasalis, Charles E., and Virginia S. Cowart. *The Steroids Game.* Champaign, IL: Human Kinetics Publishers, Inc., 1998.

Articles, Websites, and Organizations:

Ambrose, Peter J. "Doping Control in Sports—A Perspective From the 1996 Olympic Games." *American Journal of Health System Pharmacy* 54(9) (1997): 1053–1057.

Angier, Natalie. "Drugs, Sports, Body Image and G.I. Joe." *Science and Health*: December 22, 1998.

Australian Centre of Excellence in Male Reproductive Health. "Andrology Australia." Available online at *http://www.andrologyaustralia.org.*

Australian Sports Drug Agency (ASDA). "The History of Drug Use In Sport." Available online at *http://www.ausport.gov.au/fulltext/2001/asda/drugsinsporthistory.asp.*

———. "Why Do Athletes Use Drugs?" Available online at *http://www.ausport.gov.au/fulltext/2001/asda/whydo.asp.*

Bibliography

Beckham, Darren. "Blood Doping: Is it Worth It?" Available online at *http://is.tc.cc.tx.us/~mstorey/beckham.html*.

Bird, Patrick J. "Blood Doping and Erythropoietin." University of Florida, 1999. Available online at *http://www.hhp.ufl.edu/keepingfit/ARTICLE/doping&EPO.HTM*.

Brunker, Peter. *Drugs in Sport.* Speech given to the Royal Society of Victoria, October 11, 2001.

Catlin, Don, and Thomas H. Murray. "Performance-Enhancing Drugs, Fair Competition, and Olympic Sport." *Journal of the American Medical Association* 276(3)(1996): 231–237.

Dawson, Robert T. "The War on Drugs in Sport." *BMC News and Views*, 2000.

Donegan, Lawrence. "Suspicion Clouds Balco Games." *Guardian* (July 9, 2004). Available online at *http://sport.guardian.co.uk/athletics/story/0,10082,1257328,00.html*.

Dotinga, Randy. "Performance Boosting Goes Back to Ancient Olympics." *Health On the Net Foundation.* Available online at *http://www.hon.ch/News/HSN/510242.html*.

Drape, Joe. "McGwire Admits Taking Controversial Substance." *New York Times* (August 22, 1998).

Drug Enforcement Administration. "DEA Eliminates Major Source of US Meth." Available online at *http://www.usdoj.gov/dea/*.

The Economist.com. "The Secret Steroid." October 23, 2003. Available online at *http://www.economist.com/cities/PrinterFriendly.cfm?Story_ID=2156208*.

Gareau, Raynald, Michel Audran, Roy D. Baynes, Carol H. Flowers, Alain Duvallet, Louis Senecal, and Guy R. Brisson. "Erythropoietin Abuse In Athletes." *Nature* 380 (1996): 113.

Goldberg, Linn, David P. MacKinnon, Diane L. Elliot, Esther L. Moe, Greg Clarke, and JeeWon Cheong. "The Adolescents Training and Learning to Avoid Steroid Program: Preventing Drug Use and Promoting Health Behaviors." *Pediatrics and Adolescent Medicine* 154(4)(2000): 332–338.

Grandjean, Ann C. "Dietary Supplements and Athletics." *Current Opinion in Orthopedics* 13(2002): 122–127.

High Altitude Medicine Guide. "Hyperbaric Treatment—The Gamow Bag." Available online at *http://www.high-altitude-medicine.com/hyperbaric.html*.

"How Stuff Works." Available online at *http://howstuffworks.com*.

Jacobs, Ira, Harley Pasternak, and Douglas Bell. "Effects of Ephedrine, Caffeine, and Their Combination on Muscular Endurance." *The American College of Sports Medicine* 35(6)(2003): 987–994.

Johnston, Lloyd D., Patrick M. O'Malley, Jerald G. Bachman, and John E. Schulenberg. "Overview of Key Findings 2003." *Monitoring the Future—National Results on Adolescent Drug Use.* National Institute of Health Publication, 2003. Available online at *http://www.monitoringthefuture.org/pubs/monographs/overview2003.pdf.*

Knight, Jonathan. "Drug Bust Reveals Athletes' Secret Steroid." *Nature* 425(6960)(2003): 752.

Lawrence, Marvin E., and Donald F. Kirby. "Nutrition and Sports Supplements: Fact or Fiction." *Journal of Clinical Gastroenterology* 34(2002): 299–306.

Lee, Richard. "Addressing Pain: The Strategy of Medication." *Pharmacoeconomics* 3(4)(2001). Available online at *http://www.orthopedictechreview.com/issues/julaug01/pg18.htm.*

"Legal in Baseball, McGwire Uses Nutritional Supplement Banned in NFL." CNN Sports Illustrated/Associated Press. August 22, 1998. Available online at *http://sportsillustrated.cnn.com/baseball/mlb/news/1998/08/22/mcgwire_supplement/.*

Longman, Jere. *Edge Is All to Athletes, Balco Case Reveals.* June 11, 2004.

Lund, B. C., and P. J. Perry. "Non-steroid Performance Enhancing Agents in Athletic Competition: An Overview for Clinicians." *Pharmacotherapy* 2000.

Mandell, A. J., K. D. Stewart, and P. V. Russo. "The Sunday Syndrome: From Kinetics To Altered Consciousness." *Federation Proceedings* 40(1981): 2693–2968.

Mayo Clinic. "Teen Athletes And Performance-Enhancing Substances: What Parents Can Do." Available online at *http://www.mayoclinic.com/invoke.cfm?id=SM00045.*

The Medical Letter. "Performance-Enhancing Drugs." New Rochelle, NY: The Medical Letter, Inc. Vol. 46 (Issue 1187) July 19, 2004.

Nemours Foundation. "KidsHealth." Available online at *http://kidshealth.org.*

Neuroscience for Kids. "Making Connections—The Synapse." Available online at *http://faculty.washington.edu/chudler/synapse.html.*

Papazian, Ruth. "On the Teen Scene: Should You Go on a Diet." *FDA Consumer Magazine* (September 1993). Available online at *http://www.fda.gov/fdac/reprints/ots_diet.html.*

Pipe, Andrew. "Nutritional Supplements and Doping." *Clinical Journal of Sport Medicine* 12(4)(2002): 245–249.

Rannazzisi, Joseph T. DEA Congressional Testimony. March 16, 2004.

Bibliography

Reaney, Patricia. "Ancient Athletes Knew Performance-Enhancing Tricks." *Rediff.com*. Available online at *http://www.rediff.com/sports/2002/nov/14drug.htm*.

Rendell, Matt. "The Long, Lonely Road to Oblivion." *The Observer* (March 7, 2004). Available online at *http://observer.guardian.co.uk/osm/story/0,6903,1161002,00.html*.

ScienceMuseum.org. "Performance Enhancers." Available online at *http://www.sciencemuseum.org.uk/exhibitions/sport/site/education/Performanceenhancers.pdf*.

Sports-Drugs.com. Available online at *http://www.sports-drugs.com/asp/ss_features.asp*.

Stein, Rob. "Alternative Remedies Gaining Popularity—Majority in U.S. Try Some Form, Survey Finds." *Washington Post* (May 28, 2004).

Wagner, Jon C. *Stimulants and Performance*. Omaha, NE: University of Nebraska Medical Center, College of Pharmacy.

Weintraub, Arlene. "Can Drug-Busters Beat New Steroids?" *BusinessWeek* (June 14, 2004): 82.

Whyfiles.org. *Steering for Steroids*. Available online at *http://whyfiles.org/090doping_sport/3.html*.

World Anti-Doping Agency. Available online at *http://www.wada-ama.org/en/t1.asp*.

Yasalis, Charles E., Camille K. Barsukiewicz, Andrea N. Kopstein, and Micheal S. Bahrke. "Trends in Anabolic-Androgenic Steroid Use Among Adolescents." *Pediatrics and Adolescent Medicine* 151(12)(1997): 1197–1206.

Yorck, Olaf, and Ashenden M. Shumacher. "Doping with Artificial Oxygen Carriers: An Update." *Sports Medicine* 34(3)(2004): 141–150.

Further Reading

Critical Thinking:

Houlihan, Barrie. *Dying to Win—Doping in Sport and the Development of Anti-doping Policy.* Strasbourg: Council of Europe Publishing, 1999.

Stewart, Gail. *Drugs and Sports.* San Diego: Greenhaven Press, 1998.

More Facts:

Kuhn, Cynthia, Scott Swartzwelder, and Wilkie Wilson. *Pumped: Straight Facts for Athletes about Drugs, Supplements and Training.* New York: W.W. Norton & Company, Inc., 2000.

Specific Sports:

Abt, Samuel. *In Pursuit of the Yellow Jersey: Bicycle Racing in the Year of the Tortured Tour.* San Francisco: Van Der Plas Publications, 1999.

Courson, Steve. *False Glory: Steelers and Steroids: The Steve Courson Story.* Longmeadow Press, 1991.

Anabolic Androgenic Steroids:

Yesalis, Charles. *Anabolic Steroids in Sport and Exercise.* Champaign, IL: Human Kinetics Publishers, 2000.

Amphetamine:

Grinspoon, Lester. *Speed Culture: Amphetamine Use and Abuse in America.* Cambridge, MA: Harvard University Press, 1976.

An Inside Look:

Ungerleider, Steven. *Faust's Gold: Inside the East German Doping Machine.* New York: Thomas Dunne Books, 2001.

Goldman, Bob, Patricia Bush, and Ronald Klatz. *Death in the Locker Room: Steroids and Sports.* South Bend, IN: Icarus Press, 1984.

———. *Death in the Locker Room: Steroids, Cocaine and Sports.* Tucson, AZ: Body Press, 1987.

Goldman, Bob, and Ronald Klatz. *Death in the Locker Room II: Drugs and Sports in the Locker Room.* Elite Sports Publications, Inc., 1992.

Fiction:

Choyce, Lesley. *Roid Rage.* Harbour Publishing, 1999.

Websites

BBC Sports News
http://news.bbc.co.uk/sport1/hi/in_depth/2000/drugs_in_sport/default.stm

Centers for Disease Control and Prevention
www.cdc.gov/health/adolescent.htm

Drug Enforcement Administration
www.usdoj.gov/dea/

Freevibe.com
www.freevibe.com

Freudenrich, Craig. *How Performance-Enhancing Drugs Work.*
How Stuff Works
http://entertainment.howstuffworks.com/athletic-drug-test.htm

International Association of Athletics Federations
www.iaaf.org/antidoping/index.html

KidsHealth.org
http://kidshealth.org/

Monitoring the Future (survey results)
www.monitoringthefuture.org

National Institute on Drug Abuse
www.nida.nih.gov/

Office of National Drug Control Policy
www.whitehousedrugpolicy.gov

Olympics
www.olympic.org

Teendrugabuse.gov
www.teens.drugabuse.gov

United States Anti-Doping Agency
www.usantidoping.org

United States Food and Drug Administration
www.fda.gov

World Anti-Doping Agency
www.wada-ama.org/en/t1.asp

The 2004 World Anti-Doping Code
www.wada-ama.org/docs/web/standards_harmonization/
code/list_standard_2004.pdf

Index

Index

Index

Picture Credits

About the Author

Born in Langhorne, Pennsylvania, **Thomas M. Santella** holds a Bachelor's degree in Secondary English Education and is pursuing a Master of History degree at Temple University. Combining a love of knowledge and discovery with a passion for writing, he has found many opportunities to work with young people in both formal and informal educational settings. Thomas is also the Research Coordinator for Temple University's Center for Pharmaceutical Health Services Research, where he has collaborated with universities, governments, corporations, and aid organizations on a wide variety of health- and pharmaceutical-related projects. He has published work in many journals, including *The Journal of Applied Research* and *The Journal of the American Pharmacists Association*, is a freelance writer, and has traveled abroad to work on historical restoration projects such as the Benjamin Franklin House in London, England. In addition to writing and research, Santella loves traveling, hiking, reading, and music. He currently resides in Philadelphia, Pennsylvania.

About the Editor

David J. Triggle is a University Professor and a Distinguished Professor in the School of Pharmacy and Pharmaceutical Sciences at the State University of New York at Buffalo. He studied in the United Kingdom and earned his B.Sc. degree in Chemistry from the University of Southampton and a Ph.D. degree in Chemistry at the University of Hull. Following post-doctoral work at the University of Ottawa in Canada and the University of London in the United Kingdom, he assumed a position at the School of Pharmacy at Buffalo. He served as Chairman of the Department of Biochemical Pharmacology from 1971 to 1985 and as Dean of the School of Pharmacy from 1985 to 1995. From 1995 to 2001 he served as the Dean of the Graduate School, and as the University Provost from 2000 to 2001. He is the author of several books dealing with the chemical pharmacology of the autonomic nervous system and drug-receptor interactions, some 400 scientific publications, and has delivered over 1,000 lectures worldwide on his research.